Contraception

Pregnancy Prevention Using Modern Methods of Birth Control

Henrietta Blakely

Disclaimer: This book is meant to inform and empower those of whom possess a uterus. It is NOT meant to replace a conversation with a licensed healthcare provider who is familiar with the individual's complex medical history. Neither the publisher nor the author is engaged in rendering professional advice or services to the reader. The ideas, suggestions, and procedures provided in this book are not intended as a substitute for seeking professional guidance.

Contents

Introduction   vii

1. BASICS OF CONCEPTION   1
Key takeaways   5

2. A BRIEF HISTORY OF BIRTH CONTROL   7
Early history and the dangers   7
Moving towards modern solutions   9
The pill, IUDs, and birth control today   10
Stigmas that remain   12
Key takeaways   14

3. BIRTH CONTROL PILLS   15
How do birth control pills work?   15
Different hormones and their jobs   16
Different options—combination pills   17
Different options—progestin-only pills   20
Key takeaways   21

4. INTRAUTERINE DEVICES AND IMPLANTS   23
The hormonal IUD   24
The copper IUD (ParaGard)   27
Can IUDs be used as emergency contraception?   28
How to prepare and what to expect from the
procedure   28
How can you tell if your IUD moved?   30
Hormonal implant (Nexplanon)   32
Key takeaways   33

5. THE BIRTH CONTROL SHOT   35
Key takeaways   38

6. THE PATCH   39
Key takeaways   43

7. THE BIRTH CONTROL RING 45
The NuvaRing 46
The Annovera ring 47
Proper usage and insertion 48
Benefits 49
Drawbacks and side effects 50
Key takeaways 50

8. CONDOMS AND DENTAL DAMS 52
External or "male" condoms 52
Internal or "female" condoms 55
What is a dental dam? 57
Key takeaways 58

9. THE DIAPHRAGM AND THE CERVICAL CAP 59
A brief history of the diaphragm 59
How does a diaphragm work? 60
What is a cervical cap? 62
Difficulties with diaphragms and cervical caps 64
Key takeaways 65

10. THE SPONGE 66
Key takeaways 70

11. TOPICAL AGENTS 71
Spermicide 71
Vaginal acidifying gel 75
Key takeaways 76

12. PERMANENT CONTRACEPTION AND
STERILIZATION 77
Tubal ligation and female sterilization 77
Risks of tubal ligation 78
How to prepare and what to expect from the
operation 79
Vasectomies and male sterilization 80
Risks and side effects 81
Misconceptions and unfounded claims
surrounding vasectomies 81
Key takeaways 83

13. EMERGENCY CONTRACEPTION   84
What is emergency contraception?   84
Plan B and the morning-after pill   85
Ella   86
IUDs as emergency contraception   87
Key takeaways   88

14. A BRIEF SUMMARY OF NATURAL
    CONTRACEPTION   90
Natural family planning and fertility awareness   90
Lactational Amenorrhea   93
The pull-out method   94
Herbs   95
Key takeaways   97

15. OUTERCOURSE   99
What is outercourse?   99
Benefits of outercourse   100
Associated risks of outercourse   101
Key takeaways   101

16. THINGS THAT DON'T WORK   103
Key takeaways   105

Final Words   107
References   109

Introduction

Imagine this: you missed your period. *Wait a few more days,* you think to yourself. So you do. When it still doesn't come, you buy the test, the cheapest one you can find. Just something to ease your mind and tell you that you aren't pregnant.

Now you're sitting alone in your bathroom staring blankly at the positive pregnancy test. You can't believe your eyes and run to the store to buy another, it too confirms that you are pregnant. You did everything you were told but still came the unwanted and unexpected pregnancy.

From here you have to decide which unplanned pregnancy option is best for you, all of which will affect you for the rest of your life, whether it be physically or emotionally. Becoming pregnant by accident can certainly be a blessing, but more often than not, it can mean facing judgment from family, friends, and strangers on top of a strained relationship with the baby's father.

Even more, growing this life inside you will forever change your body. That is something important to consider, especially if your career is physical in nature. You may have to put your career, education, and life goals on hold for a while, and you may not be able to provide the life you wanted for your child. This change in life trajectory can be wonderful, but when the time is right. Needless to say, for better or worse, unplanned pregnancies change everything.

It's normal to have no clue what your next step is going to be, and the harsh reality is that all of this stress cannot be avoided unless you prevent the pregnancy entirely. If you choose to continue your pregnancy, you will experience the physical effects of pregnancy as well as the strain of childbirth. If you choose to terminate, the emotional stress will probably affect you for years to come. Regardless of the path you choose to take, an unwanted and unplanned pregnancy will have lifelong consequences.

The good news here is that effective birth control methods have been created and discovered, and there are options that *really* work. In this modern era, you have more access than ever to planning pregnancy, preventing it, and deciding when the time is right for you to have a child. All of which is so empowering and exciting!

I do not know your particular situation, but I do know that if more women were aware of the options and resources available, there would be a lot less stress and a lot fewer unplanned pregnancies. Knowledge is power in every aspect and can really change the course of your entire life, whether it be for lack of knowledge or access to it.

I have worked in healthcare since 2010 and have been honored to see the modern evolution of birth control methods. I have seen them change lives and people's chances of creating better futures. Furthermore, I have personally experienced the usefulness of these solutions, having used natural and prescription birth control methods throughout my life.

People who have control of how, when, and *if* they get pregnant have better health (mentally and physically), as well as better financial and social outcomes. By knowing how to prevent pregnancy when you are not ready you can create the life that is best for you now, and in the future.

There are so many methods of birth control these days, some of which are proven to be much more effective than others. In fact, there are pregnancy prevention solutions that can be as effective as 99%! If used as directed, these methods will be able to greatly reduce the chances of an unwanted pregnancy.

Spermicide and fertility-based awareness methods typically have 18 women out of 100 who get pregnant each year. Whereas birth control injections, pills, patches, and rings have 5 to 12 women out of 100. Further, an implant, IUD, or sterilization have less than one percent per year. There are so many options, and when used properly, the success rates go up!

As I am writing this, and one reason I was inspired to do so, federal legislation in the United States has decreased access to pregnancy termination. This book is not meant to be political, but this recent change will mean that the need for proper education surrounding pregnancy prevention is now more important than ever.

Access, along with real, tangible knowledge of birth control methods, provides people with control over their bodies and choices for their future. I have seen the beauty and need of these solutions, and how not being at the mercy of the choices of others is so freeing!

From pills to implants and female condoms, there are so many choices. While that is such an amazing thing and you can really choose what is best for your body, it can be overwhelming at times. I am here today to tell you that you don't need to be overwhelmed by the choices, but excited by them.

This book is a crash course in all things birth control-related, but it is not meant to replace professional help in any way. I am here to empower those with a uterus to discover more about themselves and the choices available to them. After gathering the information provided, you should have a conversation with a licensed healthcare professional who can cater to your exact needs and complex medical history.

My one hope for you now is that you will leave feeling inspired, encouraged, and in control of your body and choices. You have the power to prevent pregnancy; the tools are out there, and it's time to discover them!

Chapter 1
Basics of Conception

Understanding the basics of conception and birth control starts with understanding your menstrual cycle. You may already have a good basic idea of the general factors of menstruation, but there are actually a lot of moving parts in the menstrual cycle. So here I will go over a simple refresher along with breaking down the hormones behind it all.

On average, the menstrual cycle lasts about 28 days but can range between 20 and 40 days depending on the person, their age, how long they have been menstruating, and any health conditions they may have. This cycle is a series of changes that the female body goes through monthly to prepare for conception.

Every month, one ovary releases an egg, and this process is called ovulation. Around the same time, the body releases hormones and the uterus prepares for pregnancy. If the egg is released and is not fertilized, then it does not implant into the thickened uterine lining. Without a fertilized egg, the lining sheds through the vagina, this is called the menstrual period.

All of this is controlled by hormones and also by signals in your brain. There are two hormonal phases of your cycle, now let's look at the different hormones and what is going on inside your body each month.

The first phase is called the follicular phase, which begins on the first day of your menstrual period and ends when you ovulate. This phase varies from person to person and can last between 7 and 40 days.

The second phase of the menstrual cycle is called the luteal phase and begins when the follicular phase ends, the day of ovulation, lasting until the next period starts. Typically, this phase lasts between 12 and 16 days. Now that you know the basics of each phase, let's dive into the hormones that are controlling each piece throughout your cycle.

There's a structure in your brain called the hypothalamus, and this is where it all begins. This is a very powerful, influential, and important structure since it controls things like hunger and thirst, mood, body temperature, sex drive, sleep, and blood pressure. It also is what produces the gonadotropin-releasing hormone, or GnRH. When this hormone is produced, GnRH communicates to your pituitary gland that it is time to release the follicle-stimulating hormone (FSH). The job of FSH is to stimulate the growth and development of an egg.

The follicle-stimulating hormone will then go through your bloodstream and to your ovaries. When it arrives, it triggers a follicle's growth (a follicle being a small sac that contains the egg) and tells it to mature fully into a ready egg.

When the follicle matures, it produces the hormone called estrogen. Over the course of about ten days, estrogen levels continue to increase and peak about one day before ovulation. Meaning that in a 28-day cycle, this will typically be day 13. This spike and peak in estrogen tell your brain that the egg has fully developed and triggers the pituitary gland, which releases luteinizing hormone (LH) in a surge. This surge is basically a cue for the ovarian follicle. Within about a day, the ready egg leaves the ovary and empty follicle (or the corpus luteum) and goes into the fallopian tube where it waits for fertilization. This is what we call ovulation.

From here, your body moves onto the second phase, called the Luteal phase. Now the cells of the empty follicle sac, or the corpus luteum, will release the hormone called progesterone. This hormone causes and helps your uterine lining to thicken and prepare for implantation by a fertilized egg. For 12 to 16 days, the corpus luteum will release progesterone, all throughout the Luteal phase.

After ovulation, one of two things will happen. Either the egg is fertilized, or it is not. If your egg is fertilized, the corpus luteum will continue to produce progesterone in order to sustain the pregnancy until the placenta can take over. The placenta is an organ that is created during pregnancy to nourish the growing baby that is also expelled during childbirth. Moving back, after fertilization, the egg that has connected with the sperm will move down to the uterus and attach to the uterine lining.

The other thing that could happen is your egg isn't fertilized. In this case, the corpus luteum will begin to shrink and stop producing the hormones that would support pregnancy and the uterine lining. Now is when the lining will shed off and this leads to the start of your monthly menstrual period.

The low levels of progesterone and estrogen will tell the hypothalamus in the brain that it is time to start the whole menstrual cycle process again.

Understanding the menstrual cycle and period is one thing, but knowing if yours is normal is an entirely different animal. In fact, a lot of women are likely asking the same questions as you. *How long should my period last? How long should my cycle be? How should I track my menstrual period? Am I normal?*

As I mentioned, 28 days is about the average, but there is room for fluctuation. If you are interested in tracking your period and menstrual cycle, it is determined by starting counting on the first day of the menstrual period and continuing on until your next period starts. Your menstrual period may last two to seven days, again depending on the body. Tracking your period doesn't just mean tracking the length of your cycle, make sure to note down the length of your period, how heavy your flow is, abnormal bleeding between periods, any pain or discomfort, along with other changes.

It is also important to note that certain forms of contraception, such as IUDs (intrauterine devices) and extended-cycle birth control pills will probably alter your cycle. Be sure to talk to your doctor about what you should expect.

Irregular periods and cycles are pretty common, but there are some things that can change your cycle and even stop them from occurring. These include eating disorders, excessive exercising, extreme weight loss, polycystic ovarian syndrome (PCOS), premature ovarian failure, and uterine fibroids.

If your periods are extremely or abnormally irregular, and you miss months of bleeding, reach out to a doctor and get a professional opinion. Periods and menstrual cycles come in all shapes, colors, and sizes, and even little variables in yours can change different aspects of your cycle. But regardless of it being normal to be "abnormal", if you feel you need to talk to a doctor, do not hesitate.

Seek out professional help if you experience any of the following:

- Your cycle and bleeding is extremely irregular or excessively painful.
- Your period stops suddenly for more than 90 days, and you are not pregnant.
- Your periods suddenly become erratic and unpredictable after having been regular.
- You bleed extremely heavily or go through more than one pad or tampon in an hour or two.

- You experience bleeding between periods.
- You develop or experience severe pain or cramping during your period.

Now another question you may have: *what can I do to make my periods more regular?*

The answer here is not simple, because there are so many factors playing into your cycle and its regularity. At-home solutions won't be a surefire way of making your cycle more predictable since you don't know the root causes of it. Some women take birth control pills to help regulate their cycle, but sometimes the underlying causes cannot be prevented or treated.

Lifestyle factors also affect your period and menstrual cycle, some other things you can do holistically and within your day-to-day life include: practicing yoga, maintaining a healthy weight (being underweight can make you lose your period completely), talking to a doctor about the right daily vitamins and minerals, and getting enough physical exercise.

Key takeaways

- The menstrual cycle is not just a period of ovulation, it is a complex monthly cycle your body goes through to prepare for pregnancy.
- This cycle is controlled by hormones that trigger different reactions to begin.
- There are two phases: the follicular phase (which starts on the first day of your period and ends when you ovulate) and the luteal phase (which starts when you ovulate and ends on the first day of your next period).
- Irregular periods can be normal, and cycles fluctuate from person to person but reach out for professional help if you have concerns.

Your menstrual cycle is the beginning of it all, it is the process in charge of how and *when* you can get pregnant. Understanding birth control and discovering the effectiveness of each amazing modern method starts with a good foundational understanding of your monthly cycle. But in order to appreciate and understand these modern solutions, we should look at the history of birth control and some stigmas and unsafe methods that have plagued women through the years.

Chapter 2
A Brief History of Birth Control

Birth control pills and hormonal devices for contraception are very modern solutions, but this does not mean that other forms of birth control were not around before. In fact, contraception methods have been around for thousands of years. Thankfully, women today have access and the resources to learn more about their bodies, birth control methods, and what is actually safe.

Women throughout the ages have tried herbs, oils, plants, and other at-home remedies as contraception. Whether or not these methods were safe, one thing remains true: birth control is a necessity. As much as people will tell you to "just not have sex" or use the withdrawal method because that's what our ancestors used, it simply isn't the best option. There has always been a need for these forms of contraception, it just took a while for science and society to get to a place of embracing change and stepping into the future.

Early history and the dangers

Some of the earliest forms of contraception, as well as abortion, date back to ancient Mesopotamia and Egypt (around 1850 B.C.E). Ancient scrolls of papyrus have been found with instructions on how to make a form of birth control out of honey, lint, and acacia leaves creating a type of cervical cap to prevent sperm from impregnating the woman. In ancient Egypt, they would also use extended breastfeeding (for as long as three years) as another way of preventing pregnancy.

One of the most famous ancient forms of birth control, popular with the Greeks and Romans, is the silphium plant which is originally from North Africa. But in ancient Greece (around 1200 B.C.E) many other plants were used as forms of contraception, some of which are still used in modern medicine and birth control today (such as Queen Anne's Lace).

But overall, the most popular ancient and early form of birth control was the pull-out or withdrawal method. Even if used properly and consistently, this way of preventing fertilization is not the most effective, even today, which really gives some insight into how great the other options were.

In the Middle Ages, abortion and any form of contraception was considered immoral and the work of witches by the Catholic church. Though this did not stop many women from experimenting with plants that could block sperm, herbs to prevent pregnancy, and even concoctions that would induce a miscarriage.

In the Renaissance, barrier methods like condoms were introduced. But rather than their primary role being for birth control, they were used typically as a way to prevent the spread of Syphilis, which is a sexually transmitted infection (or STI). These were imperative because of the outbreaks across Europe and were not used as a primary form of pregnancy prevention until the early 1600s.

Long before the European settlers arrived in the Americas it was common practice among indigenous women to use herbs and plants as birth control. These included black cohosh, blue cohosh, stoneseed, thistles, and false hellebore. They were also quite aware of their menstrual cycles and could often tell when they were most or least likely to get pregnant. The natives shared these birth control methods with the Europeans, and many of them were revolutionary if not scandalous. At the time in Europe, they really had very little knowledge of contraception options outside of charms and amulets, along with practices like outercourse (or non-penetrative sexual acts). The herbal remedies and other types of birth control were actually banned widely across Europe which greatly limited their access to knowledge of family planning.

Not only were many of these early solutions highly ineffective, but a lot of them were also toxic and potentially very dangerous. One example of this is ancient Greece, where women were instructed to consume copper salt dissolved in water in order to prevent conception for up to a year… copper salt taken in this manner is highly toxic. But since childbirth and pregnancy killed so many women in history, it is no wonder why they took the risk of these birth control methods.

In the early 1800s, the United States had one of the highest birth rates in the world, with each woman birthing around eight children. At this time, just like what had been happening in Europe for so long, political and religious organizations discouraged the use of contraceptive methods and family planning, deeming them as immoral. By the early 1840s, many state governments banned the use and sale of birth control solutions, and in 1873 the federal government prohibited the sale of all contraceptives. Then, in 1888, abortion was outlawed. But throughout the mid-1800s, many people still used condoms or spermicide options along with the withdrawal method as a way of preventing pregnancy. Though many of these home remedies were still not safe.

Moving towards modern solutions

In 1909, the first IUD (intrauterine device) was created, it was a ring made of silkworm guts that was placed into the uterus. It further spread throughout Europe in the 1920s. Meanwhile, in the United States, bans surrounding contraception and sexual health education made it difficult for doctors to share these findings and new family planning information.

Around 1914 is when Margaret Sanger coined the term "birth control" bringing the term along with further education into the mainstream. She then opened the very first birth control clinic in 1916, but because of the Comstock Act (which deemed contraception terms as indecent and immoral and banned them from being published in the mail or media), it was shut down just nine days later.

When the clinic was shut down, Margaret Sanger was arrested and put on trial. This trial, and the coverage of it, sparked a revolution within the realms of sexual education and birth control. The work of Sanger and other feminist supporters, donors, and doctors started a movement intended on separating sex from procreation and making birth control widely available.

Between the 1920s and the 1950s, the media and peoples' attitudes toward birth control and sex education shifted in dramatic ways. Although the topics were still divisive, they started conversations and revolutionized the United States and many doctors' and people's views on birth control. People began questioning the government's role in family planning, sexual morality, and personal freedoms.

The pill, IUDs, and birth control today

The first ever birth control pills were created in the 1950s by Planned Parenthood Federation of America, John Rock, and Gregory Pincus. Although they were created in the 50s, the pills did not become widely available to the public until the 1960s, when it was approved by the US Food and Drug Administration (FDA) as a contraceptive. In the meantime, the ban on the use of contraceptives for married couples was officially overturned in the

Supreme Court case Griswold v. Connecticut in 1965. Another landmark step in the movement of birth control that happened in the mid-1960s was the IUD becoming available in the United States. By the late 60s, millions of people were using the pill worldwide and multiple other brands became available.

When 1972 rolled around, the ban on contraceptive use for unmarried individuals was also lifted. Later in the 70s, with technology developing rather rapidly, especially surrounding the uses of birth control, fiber optic technology was offering safer procedures and quicker recovery. Tubal ligation (or getting one's "tubes tied") was then being encouraged as a permanent form of birth control.

The 1980s and 90s were a quick-paced and revolutionary time in the world of contraception, with many new, safer forms of birth control being introduced and approved by the FDA. In 1984, the World Health Organization (WHO) approved Norplant, which is a birth control implant that only needs a single outpatient surgical placement. Norplant was not approved by the FDA to be used in the United States until 1991.

In 1988, ParaGard, the copper IUD, became available in the United States. Then, in 1992, the FDA approved the first injectable form of birth control called Depo-Provera, a form of contraception lasting three months. 1998 is when the first ever emergency contraceptive pill, Preven, received FDA approval, making it widely available to the people of the United States. A year later, in 1999, Plan B (one of the most common and well-known emergency contraceptive pills still used today) was also approved for use and sale.

From here, options and evolving forms of birth control only continue to become even more widely accessible to women in the United States and worldwide. In 2000, the hormonal IUD (similar to the copper IUD, but it releases certain hormones), called Mirena, was released to the public. Just one year later, in 2001, the first hormone-based contraceptive ring that is placed in the vagina, called the NuvaRing, also got FDA approval. And a year later, in 2002, the first ever birth control patch, Ortho Evra, (which can be applied to the skin on the upper body or lower abdomen) was also approved.

In 2006, Implanon, a birth control implant, was approved and introduced to the public, but in 2010, Nexplanon replaced it as a prescription in the United States and is instead a single-rod hormonal implant which is placed in the upper arm. Again in 2010, the FDA approved yet another form of emergency contraception, Ulipristal Acetate, which is under the drug name "Ella".

Within thirty years, so many birth control options became available, so women can choose what they put in their body. This all basically means more sexual and reproductive freedom and bodily autonomy.

From implants and IUDs to pills and emergency contraception, we certainly have come a long way from using honey and leaves as birth control. Not only do women of the twenty-first century have more options, but we have safer ones as well. Access to proper birth control is life-changing and can help prevent unwanted pregnancies that, for better or worse, change lives forever.

Stigmas that remain

Whether we like it or not, the stigmas and societal dislike of birth control have remained, though it looks a lot different than it did in the 1800s. This can create a feeling of shame for the women seeking help and information about contraceptive methods. Somehow, birth control is still such a taboo topic, one that can only be fought by rewiring your own thoughts first. Contraceptives are not a sign of a woman's promiscuity and do not validate a man's masculinity.

You might hear these things from family members, friends, or people on the internet, regardless, they are not true and should be met with informed opinions.

"If you have sex before marriage, you will get pregnant and die." This is a scare tactic that many parents, grandparents, and education systems used to teach abstinence as the only form of birth control. Further from it being complete emotional blackmail, it isn't entirely accurate either. The reality is that unprotected sex doesn't automatically mean you will get pregnant (not to mention that there are new and effective methods of birth control available). And, if you do become pregnant, it does not mean that you will die. There are certainly some risks associated with carrying a baby in your womb, but they are overstated by those who adhere to this thinking. The truth is that modern medicine has made complications less likely and less deadly.

"You're a girl. You shouldn't carry condoms. That's not ladylike." Nowadays, many people see boys getting their first box of condoms as a rite of passage and a way of becoming a man. People appreciate their initiative in making the smart choice and having safe, protected sex, and preventing pregnancy. But the same is not true for girls. The truth is that no matter who you are, it is always admirable to carry condoms and practice sexual safety. Furthermore, condoms aren't just a way of preventing pregnancy, they also help to keep you from being exposed to sexually transmitted diseases and infections.

"If you're on birth control, you must sleep around a lot." Birth control is used by people who are sexually active and do not want to get pregnant. They could be married, in a relationship, have three kids, or be single, it doesn't automatically imply a certain lifestyle. What's worse is that people would judge others based on what they *think* someone's sex life is. It is a private matter, and you are entitled to keep it to yourself.

Key takeaways

- Women throughout history have always been in search of ways to prevent pregnancy, whether it be for societal, health, or simply family planning reasons.
- The need for birth control is not modern, but these amazing modern solutions have been truly revolutionary.
- There were a lot of stigmas and shame surrounding the use of birth control, and this was only made worse by the government banning it.
- A lot has changed in a brief period. Just 60 or 70 years ago there were next to no options if you could even get a prescription. Nowadays, you have the freedom to choose.

By understanding where birth control comes from and how far we have come, I hope you are able to gain more of an appreciation for the modern solutions I will cover throughout this book. You will face misunderstandings, and be told what you should or should not do with your body at many points in your life, but at the end of the day, you really have complete freedom over your choices and your body.

Chapter 3
Birth Control Pills

How do birth control pills work?

Birth control pills, also known as oral contraception, are one of the most well-known and commonly used forms of modern pregnancy prevention. When used properly and as instructed, these pills can be up to over 99% effective. They work to suppress the hormones in your body and FSH (follicle-stimulating hormone) and LH (luteinizing hormone) with estrogen and progestin.

As we learned earlier, FSH and LH are the hormones in charge of triggering the release of estrogen from the ovaries. This, in turn, causes ovulation to occur, releasing the egg from the ovary. When these hormones are suppressed, ovulation is far less likely to occur, and therefore the fertilization of the egg by a sperm cell is significantly less likely to happen. Birth control pills also thicken your cervical mucus and make it harder for fertilization to happen on the off chance that ovulation occurs.

Birth control pills are most commonly used for what the name suggests, birth control and pregnancy prevention. But they have been found to help ease menstrual symptoms, such as cramping and heavy bleeding as well. This is because birth control pills also reduce the level of prostaglandins in your body. These are substances that cause the muscles of the uterus to contract and cause cramping and pain.

With the use of birth control, in the cases of extended or continuous dosing, you will lose your period or only have it a few times each year. With the use of conventional birth control pills, you will continue to get your period each month. Each type of birth control, whether it be pills, IUDs, or implants, has its benefits and risks. Next, I will go over the different contraceptive pill options available today.

Different hormones and their jobs

In birth control, two main hormones are used; These are estrogen and progesterone (or progestin, in this case). They either work together—in combination type pills or progestin works alone in a progestin-only pill.

Progestin is the synthetic form of progesterone that is naturally found and released in the body. Progesterone is released from a woman's ovaries and helps to prepare the body for pregnancy, preventing lactation, building the uterine lining for implantation, and strengthening the pelvic walls to prepare for labor. If the egg is not fertilized, then progesterone levels drop. Naturally, in the typical menstrual cycle, progesterone acts as a trigger and aids in ovulation, but shifted levels of *progestin* actually work to stop ovulation and prevent pregnancy.

Estrogen, just like progesterone, is a natural sex hormone created by a woman's body. It is responsible for a woman developing her sex characteristics and is prominent in a girl's development through puberty. During pregnancy, estrogen works to support the functions that create and secrete breast milk. When there is estrogen in birth control (a combination pill) then it works alongside the progesterone to prevent pregnancy by making it harder for the sperm to reach the egg and consistently stopping ovulation.

Different options—combination pills

Combination birth control pills are one form of the oral contraceptive, otherwise known as Combined Estrogen-progestin Oral Contraceptives (COCs), that contain both estrogen and progestin, as the name suggests. These pills keep your ovaries from being stimulated and releasing an egg for ovulation, far more consistently than some progestin-only pills. As I mentioned earlier, they also increase cervical mucus to keep the sperm from reaching the egg if it is released. There are different options for dosing, and each has a different amount and ratio regarding estrogen and progestin levels.

There are a few options for cycles and packs of pills. The first is the conventional pack, which is the most common kind and contains 21 active pills and 7 inactive ones. With these packs, you take one pill every day and immediately start a new pack when you finish the old one, which is every 28 days. Bleeding, like a period, occurs during the last week of the pack when you take the 7 inactive pills.

Then there are the continuous dosing, or extended cycle, packs. Usually, these will contain 84 active pills and 7 inactive pills. Bleeding will typically only occur four times each year, during the weeks that you take the 7 inactive pills. There is also the option to have 365 days of the same active pill. For most women, this makes their periods stop, and for others, it just becomes a whole lot lighter. Along with suppressing periods, extended cycle packs bring along other added benefits such as reducing excessive bleeding from uterine fibroids, preventing migraines related to menstruation, and pain relief from endometriosis.

Taking these COCs can be done in a few ways other than just the cycle length. Your birth control pills mimic your menstrual cycle, therefore, starting your pills the first day of your cycle, or the first Sunday after your cycle is recommended. This is called the *Sunday start* method of syncing your birth control pills to your natural rhythms. With this method, and with most use of combined oral contraceptives, you do not need to worry about supplementing your birth control with another form of contraception.

You can also use the *any-day start* method, which means you start your pack the day you pick them up, regardless of what day of your cycle you are on. However, starting right away means it will take a while for your cycle and the hormones of the pills to sync up. Using this timing method also means that after the termination of a pregnancy or a miscarriage, you can start the pills back up immediately or whenever you want. But this is typically not recommended after childbirth, as the hormones in the pills can affect breast milk supply. So, as a general rule of thumb, you should wait at least three weeks after giving birth to start these combined oral contraceptives again, and only with the approval of your licensed healthcare provider.

Combined Oral Contraceptives, as I mentioned, contain both estrogen and progestin (or synthetic progesterone). But it's not quite as simple as that. There are many types of estrogens and progestins available. The types of estrogen found in COCs can be Estradiol, Ethinylestradiol, or Estetrol. And there are even more options for progestins. In fact, there are three different generations of progestins and unclassified progestins.

First-generation progestins include Norethindrone acetate, Ethynodiol diacetate, Lynestrenol, and Norethynodrel. Second generation progestins include Levonorgestrel and dl-Norgestrel. Third generation progestins include Norgestimate, Gestodene, and Desogestrel. Unclassified progestins include Drospirenone and Cyproterone acetate. These options can be really overwhelming, so talk to your health care professional about your needs and figure out what will be best for you.

When taking these pills, there are also different options for how the dosage fluctuates within the time you are taking them. They can be monophasic COCs, meaning they have the same dosage of hormones from start to finish in every pill (with the placebo at the end). Or they can be multiphasic COCs, which means you will have different dosages of hormones every week, again with the placebo likely at the end.

Combination pills are a very common form of birth control that is highly reliable and easily reversed, unlike some other options I will talk about later in this book. In fact, you will return to your normal fertile self relatively quickly after stopping the pills. But besides contraception, they have other non-pregnancy-related benefits as well, including (but not limited to):

- Treating and improving acne
- Decreasing the risk for ovarian and endometrial cancers
- Decreased risk for ovarian cysts
- Pain relief for menstrual cramps
- Lighter, shorter, and often more regular periods and menstrual cycles
- PMS (premenstrual syndrome) relief
- Decreased risk for benign breast disease

While these pills are great and provide many benefits, they are not suitable for those in certain situations, such as:

- Those with breast cancer
- If you are breast-feeding
- If you are pregnant... *obviously*
- If you experience certain types of migraines
- Have poorly controlled blood pressure
- Have a history of heart disease or strokes
- Experience unexplained uterine bleeding
- If you have liver disease
- You are over 35 and smoke regularly

Be sure to discuss these factors with your doctor to figure out what will work best in your case. A healthcare professional will give you more insight into what you should or should not be taking.

There are some side effects including possible interaction with vitamin and mineral supplementation, bleeding or spotting between periods, nausea, headaches, bloating, breast tenderness, and higher blood pressure.

Different options—progestin-only pills

Other than combination pills, there are progestin-only birth control pills as well, which don't contain any estrogen. In the United States, progestin-only pills (POPs) will be either Norethindrone or Drospirenone, which are different types of synthetic progesterone. In the United Kingdom, there are even more progestin-only pill options. The different progestins are naturally dosed differently, with Norethindrone being dosed at 0.35mg once every day with a 28 day pill pack, and Drospirenone being dosed at 4 mg daily for 24 days and 4 days of hormone-free, or placebo, pills per 28 day pill pack. With each of these different options, your cycle will react differently, and you will probably not know until you start. You might bleed or spot a little throughout the month, lose your period entirely, or still get your period like normal.

POPs or mini pills can be started immediately, regardless of the cycle option you choose (28 days of hormones, or a cycle where you have 4 days of hormone-free pills). For Norethindrone, you can start it any day of your cycle, but you should use another form of contraception alongside the pills for the first 48 hours. With Drospirenone (otherwise known as Slynd in the United States) you should use a backup method of birth control for the first seven days after starting.

But it is always best to discuss with a licensed healthcare professional about start dates and what their recommendations are. This is because these pills are typically most effective if started on the first day of your period, and that is the current preferred method of starting. It is also important to note that there may be a higher chance of pregnancy if you do not take the pills at the same time every day, or at least within the same three-hour window. Also, note that with progestin-only pills your fertility will also return to normal pretty much immediately after stopping use.

Additionally, due to the fact that they do not contain any estrogens, they have been deemed safe to use while breastfeeding and for individuals who may have conditions that are negatively affected by estrogens. A healthcare professional may also recommend progestin-only pills if you have other health problems such as blood clots in the lungs or legs, or if you have an increased risk for those conditions.

Avoid use if:

- You have or are at high risk of having breast cancer
- You have liver disease
- You experience unexplained and irregular uterine bleeding
- You have a changing schedule and won't be able to take the pill at the same time every day

It is also important to note that both combination and progestin-only birth control pills will interfere and, or, negatively react with certain antibiotics. It is highly recommended that you use another backup form of birth control and contraception if you are taking these pills and antibiotics simultaneously.

Key takeaways

- Birth control pills can be up to 99% effective when used properly and when prescribed the correct dosage for your body.

- There are two types of pills, combination oral birth control (which combines estrogen and progestin) and progestin-only pills (which contain no estrogen.)
- Both types work to stop ovulation and thicken your cervical mucus, which makes it harder for the sperm to reach the egg if it is released.
- Birth control pills aren't only used to prevent pregnancy, in fact, they are often used to treat things such as premenstrual syndrome (PMS) symptoms, menstrual cramping, acne, and more.
- There are different routes you can take with combination pills: the monophasic route which is all the same dosage until the placebo pills at the end, or the multiphasic route which changes the dosage of the hormones each week.
- There are also different cycle lengths you can choose and discuss with your doctor. The first is the conventional cycle which is three weeks long. The other is an extended cycle pill that can range from 84 to 365 days and will probably stop your period entirely.
- Some cautions: do not take combination birth control pills if you have breast cancer, are breastfeeding, if you are pregnant, if you experience frequent migraines, have poorly controlled blood pressure, experience unexplained uterine bleeding, if you have liver disease, or if you are over 35 and smoke regularly.
- Progestin-only pills are good for those whose bodies react poorly to estrogen supplementation, or who have a condition that is negatively affected by estrogen.
- These are more likely to be effective if they are taken at the same time (or around the same time) every day.
- Do not take progestin-only pills if you have, or you are at high risk of having, breast cancer, if you have liver disease, if you experience unexplained and irregular uterine bleeding, or if you have a changing schedule and won't be able to take the pill at the same time every day.

Chapter 4
Intrauterine Devices and Implants

We have come a long way from the 1909 version of an Intrauterine Device (IUD) that was made of silkworm guts. The early IUDs were only used for people who had previously had a baby, but now they are generally available for anyone who has a uterus. Nowadays, these implants and intrauterine devices are so high-tech (at least compared to the previous versions) and come with different options so you can choose what is best for you and your uterus.

In basic terms, an IUD is a little device that is inserted into the uterus and can prevent pregnancy. Sometimes IUDs (intrauterine devices) are called IUCs, or intrauterine contraception, and these birth control devices are *T*-shaped pieces of plastic with a small string attached at the end. In the case of the copper intrauterine device, it is wrapped in a coil of copper and does not contain any hormones.

The hormones and the copper in these IUDs or implants work by what may seem like a miracle to the naked eye. But the reality is that the hormones in the hormonal IUD and implant and the copper in the ParaGard IUD (or copper intrauterine device) work by thinning the uterine lining, which makes it harder for the egg and the sperm to connect and implant, thickening the cervical mucus, and actually changing the way and direction sperm move in order to prevent pregnancy.

This method of birth control is long-lasting, each of the different options having a different lifespan ranging between three and twelve years. They are also over 99% effective, meaning less than one percent of women with an IUD or implant each year will get pregnant.

These devices must be inserted and typically removed by a licensed professional. Unlike with oral birth control, the insertion of these devices may cause a bit of pain, but this all depends on the woman. When they are removed, with all three options I will discuss, it is possible to become pregnant right after removal.

IUDs are supposed to be taken out by a licensed healthcare provider, though in rare instances, IUDs can come out on their own. Your healthcare provider can give you instructions on how to check for the strings against your cervix to ensure that it is still in place. If you suspect that your IUD may have come out, use a backup birth control method until you can have a healthcare provider confirm.

The hormonal IUD

Hormonal IUDs are one option for long-acting reversible contraception. They are made of flexible plastic and are usually *T-shaped*, just like the other IUDs. A hormonal IUD releases one hormone that I talked about in the previous chapter, called progestin. This bit of the hormone within the IUD is released little by little over a long period, several years actually.

The hormonal IUD is a highly effective form of contraception and is over 99% effective in preventing pregnancy. They can be left in for three to eight years depending on which IUD you choose, which makes them a great option for those who do not want to worry about maintenance or having to constantly purchase pills and condoms.

The hormonal intrauterine device is available under four different names in the United States: Mirena, Kyleena, Liletta, and Skyla. These all work the same way and have the same hormones in them. The crucial difference you will find here is the length of time for which they are effective. The Liletta and Mirena IUDs last the longest, for up to eight years. Meanwhile, Kyleena works for about five years, and Skyla has the shortest life of three years. The good thing here is that you don't *have* to keep your IUD for that many years, you can get it removed whenever you want! Further, if your IUD is going to expire and you want to keep using one, your doctor can usually remove and replace it in the same appointment.

In the United Kingdom, there are even more options for IUDs, which vary in size, hormone amounts, length of use, and even metal content. Some IUDs in the United Kingdom include gold or silver in addition to the standard copper IUD. There is also a frameless (non-T-Shaped) copper-containing IUD offered in the UK called Gynefix, which is much smaller and lasts for up to five years.

Even more than just preventing unwanted pregnancy, hormonal IUDs help improve premenstrual syndrome symptoms such as severe cramps. You may also experience lighter monthly periods, spotting on your period, or may even lose your period completely. Many people actually use these IUDs to treat other period problems. Pregnancy prevention is an added benefit. Conditions like polycystic ovarian syndrome (PCOS) and endometriosis can be incredibly painful while a person is on their period, but the hormones in these IUDs often are great at treating many of these symptoms.

Some other benefits include:

- It eliminates having to interrupt sex for the use of contraception.
- It doesn't require partner participation.

- There are no side effects attached to the hormone estrogen (since there is only progestin).
- Can be used while still breastfeeding. But it is usually advised to wait a while after childbirth so it doesn't inflame the already traumatized pelvic walls.

But the reality of birth control is that it is not always fine and dandy, and there will be downsides and side effects to every option you have. With the hormonal IUD, some people report spotting between periods, more irregular and unpredictable periods, and quite a bit of cramping after insertion. This can last approximately 3-6 months while your body gets used to it.

It is also important to note that hormonal IUDs are not for everyone. Your doctor may discourage use if you:

- Have breast cancer, or have had it in the past
- Have uterine or cervical cancer
- Experience unexplained bleeding between periods
- Have a pelvic inflammatory disease or pelvic infection
- Have uterine fibroids, as they will interfere with the insertion
- Have liver disease

There are also some side effects to consider before getting this form of birth control. These include headaches, acne, tender breasts, mood swings and changes, cramping and pelvic pain after insertion, and irregular bleeding (which usually resolves after about 3-6 months).

Also, be sure to talk to your healthcare provider in advance if you are currently taking any medications (including herbal drugs and nonprescription medicines), have heart disease or diabetes, experience migraines, have blood clotting or stroke problems, or if you have a heart condition.

The copper IUD (ParaGard)

The copper IUD, just like the hormonal one, is a small T-shaped piece of very flexible plastic with a plastic string attached at the end (which protrudes from the cervix after insertion). But rather than just being made of plastic, it is wrapped in a coil of copper. When these are inserted properly, they are over 99% effective in preventing pregnancy, and can last up to ten to twelve years, depending upon the brand.

It is inserted in the same way as the hormonal IUD, but instead of releasing hormones into your womb, it releases copper. The copper acts to thicken your cervical mucus, changes the way the sperm swim (so they can't meet the egg) and even makes it so that a fertilized egg can't implant into the uterine lining.

Once an IUD is fitted and inserted, it is effective immediately, so much so that it can act as emergency contraception (more on that later). Even better, since there are no hormones involved, pretty much anyone with a uterus can use this contraceptive method. Again, because there are no hormones in this IUD, you won't experience the hormonal side effects like you would with the hormonal options. These avoided side effects include headaches, acne, and tender breasts.

Copper IUDs are safe to use when you are breastfeeding, don't interrupt sex, and won't be affected by other medicines, supplements, or antibiotics.

But as I mentioned earlier, there are always two sides to every coin. Here are some disadvantages that come along with the copper IUD:

- It doesn't protect against sexually transmitted diseases and infections
- Your period flow may become longer, heavier, and even come with more painful cramps (though for most, this typically goes back to normal after a few months)

- It may cause spotting and bleeding between periods

Can IUDs be used as emergency contraception?

Actually, certain IUDs work well as forms of emergency contraception, and are about 99% effective in preventing pregnancy if inserted within 5 days (or 120 hours) of having unprotected sex. This is actually one of the most effective forms of emergency contraception, with some of the highest success rates.

Another significant benefit to using IUDs as emergency birth control is that you can keep it in place for many years as highly effective birth control and do not need to use other emergency contraception, like the morning-after pill.

How to prepare and what to expect from the procedure

Be sure to eat a light meal or small snack about half an hour before the procedure so that you do not get lightheaded or faint. It may also do you well to bring along a sugary drink or piece of candy if you get dizzy. Before you head in, you should also ask your doctor if you should take a pain reliever beforehand, or if they will provide something for you. This can help with some of the discomforts from the insertion and cramping that comes directly after the procedure.

Now, what should you expect from the procedure?

When you get to the office of a healthcare professional, you will be instructed to lie down on an exam table with your legs up and open. Your provider will then insert a speculum into your vagina, opening it so that they can see the cervix clearly. Some places will do an ultrasound to measure the depth of your womb beforehand, but this isn't done everywhere. When the speculum is inside your vagina, your provider will then clean your cervix and vagina with an antiseptic solution. After cleaning, they will use special instruments to check the size and position of the uterus along with lining it up with the cervix.

From here, they will prepare for the actual insertion, folding down the "arms" of the IUD and placing it into an applicator tube. This tube is then pushed up through the little opening in your cervix. When it is placed inside your womb, the applicator tube will release the arms, the IUD will open, and the applicator tube will be removed. The strings will then hang down into your vagina, and your provider will trim them so that they don't come down too far. The strings will soften and curl up over time, making them less noticeable to you and your partner.

The entire procedure lasts between five and fifteen minutes, but you may want to stay on the table for a few minutes to take a couple of breaths. Be sure to only stand up when you are fully ready. If you feel lightheaded or dizzy, sit back down and stay in the doctor's office until you feel better. This is also a great time for that sugary drink or piece of candy.

The insertion can be anxiety-inducing for some, as typically they don't know what to expect or did not anticipate any pain. For most individuals, the insertion is only slightly uncomfortable. Of course, your body is not accustomed to having anything inserted into the uterus, and as such, you may feel some cramping as your doctor inserts the IUD and directly afterward as well. It is possible that you may experience some significant pain, but it really just depends on the person. Your healthcare provider should discuss with you what kind of pain is normal and what is not. It may be best to plan for the worst and take a pain reliever at your doctor's advice.

After the procedure, you can expect to experience some mild cramping and spotting for a few days. For this cramping, you can take over-the-counter pain relief and try to use a heating pad to ease the cramps. If you begin to feel extremely severe cramps, pain, or excessive bleeding or find that it isn't getting better, contact your doctor right away.

You will also be advised to avoid penetrative sex for at least 24 hours after insertion due to possible pain, and this timeline may be longer for some people with some doctors recommending up to a week. Just don't insert anything into your vagina for at least 24 hours.

After the insertion, your doctor will teach you how to check if the strings are in place. This is something you should do monthly, and if you don't feel them or if they feel longer than before, call your doctor right away. You should also contact your doctor immediately if you think you are pregnant, have excessive bleeding on your periods, have chills or a fever over 100.4 degrees Fahrenheit (or 38 degrees Celsius), experience pain during sex, have a sharp pain in your lower stomach or pelvis, feel dizzy, or have been exposed to an STI.

How can you tell if your IUD moved?

It is rare, but there are cases of women who get an IUD and it moves out of place or even falls out entirely. The most common time for IUDs to move is during the first few months after placement. After that time period, it is far less likely to happen.

Here are some reasons why your IUD may move or fall out of place:

- You experience stronger than normal uterine contractions during your period
- Your uterus has a drastic tilt
- Your uterine cavity is small
- A doctor without proper experience inserted the IUD
- You are breastfeeding
- You are under 20 years old
- You had the IUD put in too soon after giving birth

A suction-based menstrual product, such as a menstrual cup, may also pull out an IUD if you are not careful. If you use these products, break the suction seal before removing to avoid displacing your IUD.

While these are not direct signs that your IUD *will* fall out, they may contribute to the risk of having it shift or come out. There are some things you can do to check on its placement. As I previously mentioned, IUDs have small strings that hang down through the cervix and into the vagina. Doctors recommend checking these strings once each month after your period. Here is how you can do that.

First, wash your hands with antibacterial soap and water. Now you will want to sit on a chair or the toilet or squat down, with your legs wide so that you can access your vagina. Put a finger into your vagina and push it up until you feel your cervix. Now, feel around for the ends of the strings that should hang out of your cervix. Make sure that they feel the same as they did when your IUD was newly inserted, but make sure not to tug on the strings or move them around too much.

Here are some signs that your IUD may have moved, besides the strings, feeling longer or shorter than usual:

- Being able to feel the plastic part of the IUD protruding from the cervix
- Your partner suddenly being able to feel your IUD during sex
- Bleeding between periods
- Excessively heavy period flows
- Unusual vaginal discharge
- Pain, unusual cramping, or consistent soreness in the lower abdomen
- Cramping outside of when you normally experience period cramps

If you think that your IUD may have moved, don't put it back in by yourself, call a doctor right away and let them know what you are thinking. It is better to be safe than sorry.

Hormonal implant (Nexplanon)

Nexplanon (aka the hormonal birth control implant) is a tiny, thin rod of plastic about the size of a match. Nexplanon is the modern, most recent version of this contraceptive method, but there is actually an older version called Implanon.

This implant is not inserted into your uterus like IUDs, instead, it is placed under the skin in your upper arm. It works by releasing a hormone into your body that prevents you from getting pregnant. This hormone is called progestin, and it closely resembles the naturally made progesterone in your body. This birth control is another "one and done" option since once it is inserted, you can use it and not have to worry about contraceptive methods for up to three years. It is also over 99% effective in preventing unwanted pregnancies. Not only that, but it is easily reversible, so if you decide to try to conceive later on, you can have it removed and get pregnant relatively quickly soon after removal.

The birth control implant works to prevent pregnancy in two ways: first, the progestin thickens the cervical mucus, which makes it harder for the sperm to swim to meet the egg. Second, progestin also stops the release of the egg in the first place, and no egg and no sperm means no pregnancy.

Like with all medicines and most birth control methods, there are side effects. These include:

- Changes in menstruation such as longer or shorter bleeding, spotting between periods, irregular cycles, and sometimes no bleeding at all.
- Mood swings and changes
- Weight gain

- Depressed mood
- Headaches
- Breast tenderness and pain
- Acne
- Stomach pain
- Nausea
- Dizziness
- Back pain
- Pain at the place it was inserted

These are not side effects everyone experiences, but they could affect you. It is better to be prepared for the worst rather than not be prepared at all.

The hormonal birth control implant is, once again, not for everyone. You should talk to your doctor about further information if you have any allergies, have liver disease or a tumor, experience unexplained vaginal bleeding, have or have had blood clots in the past, or if you have had breast cancer previously.

You should also remember that just because implants and IUDs are great at preventing pregnancy, they cannot protect against sexually transmitted diseases and infections. It is better to be safe than sorry and use a condom when you don't know if the person you are engaging with sexually has been tested.

Key takeaways

- Intrauterine devices are little T-shaped plastic devices that are inserted into the uterus and either contain hormones or a small metal coil that is usually made of copper.
- IUDs and implants have very high success rates if used and inserted properly.

- These birth control solutions are long term and basically mean that once you get it inserted you don't need to worry about contraception for three to twelve years.
- The copper IUD may cause cramping and heavier periods, whereas the hormonal IUD may ease cramping and lighten period flows.
- Preparing for IUD insertion might be a great option for those who are nervous about the procedure or are likely to become dizzy or faint. Be sure to eat a light meal before or bring along something that can bring your blood sugar up in case you get lightheaded.
- Implants are placed under the skin in your upper arm and only come in hormonal options that release progestin into your body to prevent unwanted pregnancy.
- Every kind of birth control, especially hormonal, regardless of how effective and innovative, will have side effects. There will never be a "one size fits all" solution, so it is up to you and your doctor to figure out what is the best option for you.
- These are not barrier methods and therefore cannot protect against sexually transmitted diseases and infections. If you are having sexual contact with someone and you are not sure if they have been tested, it is also best to use a condom.

Chapter 5
The Birth Control Shot

The birth control shot, also known as the depo-shot or Depo-Provera, is an injection you get once every 3 months from a healthcare provider as a form of pregnancy prevention. Depo-Provera (depo-medroxyprogesterone acetate, or DMPA) is an injection that is progestin-based and is a convenient form of birth control that is generally recognized as safe by the FDA. Though the birth control shot was originally developed in the 1960s, it wasn't FDA approved and widely available to the public in the United States until 1992.

It is a very convenient way of preventing pregnancy since once you get it injected, you do not need to worry about another form of contraception until it's time to get it injected again. Though it is highly important to remember when you need to get the shot again, because if you are not on time, you will have a higher chance of getting pregnant unexpectedly.

The hormone in this shot is a progestin, the synthetic form of our natural progesterone. It works to prevent ovulation from happening. When there is no egg in the tube, there can't be any pregnancy. It also thickens the cervical mucus and keeps the sperm from being able to reach the uterus. Though it is important to note that the birth control shot cannot protect against sexually transmitted diseases and infections.

The birth control shot is, as I mentioned, highly effective and convenient. When the injection is used properly, meaning you are always on time for your scheduled appointments, this form of contraception is over 99% effective. But in reality, the shot is actually closer to 94% effective, since some people forget to schedule more appointments or forget to go to them. This basically means that the better you are at getting your shot on time, the better it works.

Getting the birth control shot is also relatively simple and makes your job of remembering contraception methods even easier. After you discuss your birth control options with your doctor, if you decide on the depo-shot, you will then move on to create a schedule with them. In order for the shot to be fully effective, you need to be getting a fresh shot 4 times a year, or every three months, though this rounds out to be every 12 to 13 weeks. You and your health care provider will figure out a start date and subsequent injections together.

You can get your first birth control shot at whatever stage in your cycle. If you get it within the first seven days of your cycle, you will be protected from getting pregnant right away, and that is why health care providers typically recommend this timing. If you get it at any other time in your cycle, use another form of birth control, such as a condom, for the first seven days after having the shot. You can also have this injection as soon as five days after giving birth since it should not interfere with milk production due to it being progestin-only.

After your first injection, it is then all about remembering to set your alarms and create new appointments for the follow-up shots. You can keep track of your timing and appointments by setting alarms and reminders on your phone, marking it on the calendar, or even asking a friend or family member to remind you. If you are two or more weeks late to have your follow-up injection, your healthcare provider may ask you to take a pregnancy test or even emergency contraception if you have had unprotected vaginal sex within the last five days (or 120 hours).

While this is a highly effective form of birth control, there are some downsides and side effects. Some of the most notable drawbacks for people are the potential for weight gain and the increased risk of developing osteoporosis with prolonged use. There is also a delayed return to fertility after stopping the shot, which could actually be considered a benefit to some people.

Side effects include:

- Changes to your period, especially within the first year.
- Bleeding more than usual
- Spotting between periods—though this is completely normal and totally safe
- Not getting your period at all
- Nausea
- Headaches
- Sore breasts
- Depressed mood
- Slight bruising at the site of the injection

Do note that there is a slightly increased risk of breast cancer and endometrial cancer with the use of the depo-shot. It is important to discuss these risks with your healthcare provider prior to starting this form of birth control.

The side effects of the birth control shot typically go away completely after two to three months, or once your body gets used to the hormones. If you don't like the side effects or the way the injection makes you feel, contact your health care provider to discuss other options of birth control.

Key takeaways

- The birth control shot (also known as the depo-shot or Depo-Provera) was originally developed in the 1960s but did not receive FDA approval until 1992.
- It is a progestin-based injection that works by stopping ovulation and thickening cervical mucus so the sperm and the egg cannot meet.
- This is a highly effective form of contraception, being over 99% effective if used properly.
- If an IUD or an implant isn't the right choice for you, this is another low-maintenance form of birth control, you just need to make sure you go in for a follow-up shot every three months.
- It is important to remember your appointments for more shots since they aren't effective if you are two or more weeks late. In these cases, your doctor may have you take a pregnancy test or emergency contraception if you have had sex within the last 120 hours.
- The depo-shot does not protect against sexually transmitted infections, so consider also using a condom as discussed previously.

Chapter 6
The Patch

The birth control patch is a combined estrogen and progestin patch that is worn on the skin to reduce the incidence of unwanted pregnancy. It is generally safe, convenient, and works very well if worn properly. When you wear this patch on certain parts of the body, it can release hormones through the skin that act as your contraception. It is sticky, won't come off in water, and is applied once weekly. Currently, in the United States, there are two brands available, under the names Xulane and the Twirla patch. In the United Kingdom, it is called the Evra patch.

The contraceptive patch works to prevent pregnancy by stopping the sperm from reaching the egg, and just like a lot of other methods, the hormones in it work to mimic your natural cycles. The hormones estrogen and progestin work to stop ovulation and make it so that the sperm can't connect with an egg and implant in the uterus. Also similar to other birth controls, the progestin in the patch works to make the cervical mucus thicker, blocking the sperm from reaching the womb.

Even though it comes in quite the unconventional form, this little patch is highly effective if used properly—up to 99.4% even! There are no pills to swallow, no painful cramping or procedures, and no under-the-skin insertion.

To use the patch and make it work the best it can, you place it on your back, belly, lower abdomen, or buttocks. In order to reap the full powers of the birth control patch, correct application is key—you can't just slap it on anywhere and expect to be protected from pregnancy. Making a mistake in the application, or forgetting to get refills or replace it on time are the main reasons for women getting pregnant while using this contraceptive method. Now we'll talk about a few of the ways you can make the patch work best for you, starting with proper application instructions.

Each patch is a little different, so read the instructions and speak to a health care provider before use. First, you need to know *where* you are going to apply the patch. As I mentioned, the upper arm, back, belly, and bottom are all great locations for the patch—just double check on the instructions of your specific birth control patch to make sure all of those locations work. Now find a spot where there is not much hair and rinse it with soap and water, tapping it completely dry. From here, just stick it right on.

The contraceptive patch is to be applied on the first day of your period (and the first day of your cycle) and to be worn for seven days. Then, on day eight, remove and replace it immediately with a new patch that you can wear for another seven days. The cycle continues like this: remove and replace that patch on day 15 to wear for another seven days, then remove that patch on day 22 without replacing it, until day 28. This time off from wearing the patch should produce bleeding similar to a period. You will then replace the patch the day after day 28, this is now day 1 of your cycle.

Similarly to COCs (combined oral contraceptives), there are different cycle options. If you would prefer to skip the bleeding stage and keep continuous dosing through that week, there are options for you.

Here are some other tips to make the patch work even better for you:

- Use a reminder app or set a weekly alarm to replace your patch.
- Write down the days you are supposed to remove and replace your patch on the calendar.
- Have your partner or family member help remind you to get refills.
- Keep new and unused patches in the same place every time so that you don't lose them.
- Store your unused patches away from direct sunlight and at room temperature. Also, keep the patch sealed in its pouch until you are ready to put it on your skin.
- Apply the patch where it will not be rubbed by tight clothes, like a waistband, bra, or underwear.
- Check your patch once daily to make sure it is still applied properly and not falling off.
- If you are using Twirla, be sure to not allow it to be in water for more than 30 minutes at a time.
- Read the directions on your specific patch to make sure you know all the details, it also doesn't hurt to ask your health care provider if you have any questions at all.

The patch actually has quite a few other benefits as well. The effects that aren't just birth control in the patch aren't always a bad thing, in fact, some people don't even use the patch with its primary use as a contraceptive at all. Some health benefits and things the patch can help with include: treatment of acne, slowed progression of bone thinning, reduction of ovarian cysts, reduction of cysts in your breasts, prevention of ectopic pregnancies, prevention of ovarian and endometrial cancers, management of premenstrual syndrome (PMS) symptoms, and even reduction in iron deficiency. The patch can also make your periods lighter and less painful. It can even make your cycle more predictable if you were irregular previously.

It is possible to get pregnant right away after stopping the use of the birth control patch. Some people on birth control aren't against having babies, they just want to wait until the time is right, and with the birth control patch, women will choose when they want to try to conceive. After you stop using the patch, it can take around one to three months before your periods and menstrual cycle return to normal, but your fertility returns to normal relatively quickly. Your menstrual cycle should sync up again within a maximum of six months. However, if your periods were irregular before, this timeline can be quite a bit longer than normal.

Also, since your patch is already working and active for a full week, that means you don't need to interrupt the flow of sex to grab a condom or other form of contraception. This means you have pregnancy protection for as long as you are wearing the active patch. But please note that birth control patches do not protect you from sexually transmitted diseases and infections, so wearing a condom for those purposes is always wise if you don't know the status of your partner.

In order to get the birth control patch, you actually need a prescription. You can get this prescription from a doctor or nurse at a doctor's office, a health clinic, or a local Planned Parenthood center (in the United States). During your visit to your health care provider, you will discuss your concerns and medical history and your doctor or nurse will check your vital signs (temperature, blood pressure, heart rate, and respirations). Depending on the person, this patch could be the right option or not, but this is entirely up to you and your doctor. Immediately after receiving a prescription, you can get the patches from your doctor or be given a note to pick them up from your local drugstore or pharmacy.

But with every amazing and innovative form of contraception, there are always downsides and side effects. One of the biggest drawbacks is that if you aren't able to replace the patch on time, your birth control will not be active, so if you struggle with remembering things on a weekly basis, this method may not be for you.

Many people who use the patch experience no problems at all, others can experience a few issues, it all depends from person to person.

Side effects and risks include the following:

- Bleeding or spotting between periods
- Breast tenderness
- Nausea
- Headaches
- And an increased risk for blood clots

Please note that these side effects generally go away within two to three months of use, as your body gets used to the hormones in the patch. But you should not feel sick or uncomfortable with this form of birth control. The good news here is that you have so many options available to you, so if this isn't the right one for you, there are tons of others you can try.

If you are someone who experiences migraine with aura, it is not recommended for you to use the birth control patch as it increases your risk of having a stroke. As always, your healthcare provider is the best resource to determine if this method is safe for you.

Key takeaways

- The patch is a very convenient form of birth control and only needs to be replaced once every seven days, not every time you have sex.
- The patch is a hormonal form of birth control containing estrogen and progestin, working to prevent pregnancy in a similar way to combined oral contraceptives.
- Proper application is key: apply to the right area, within reach, and to clean, dry, and relatively hairless skin.
- It is also a highly effective way to prevent pregnancy, with effectiveness up to 99% when used correctly.

- Tracking your cycle days can be hard, but setting reminders and counting on the calendar can make it a lot easier.
- The contraceptive patch has a lot of other benefits as well, including lighter and less painful periods, less acne, helping with iron deficiency, and making your PMS symptoms better.
- But there are some side effects that include: spotting between periods, tender breasts, headaches, nausea, and an increased risk for blood clots.
- The birth control patch does not protect against sexually transmitted diseases and infections, so consider also using a barrier method if you do not know the status of your partner.

Chapter 7
The Birth Control Ring

The birth control ring, also known as the vaginal ring or "the ring", is a small and flexible ring that you wear inside the vagina. It is simple, easy, and convenient and works by releasing hormones into your body throughout the day, protecting you from pregnancy. There are two different kinds of birth control rings, the NuvaRing and Annovera. As always, this highly effective form of contraception is only effective if worn and used properly. If used correctly, the birth control ring is 99% effective, but people aren't perfect, and allowing for mistakes, that number drops to 91%.

Each ring has a different life span and way of use, you just need to make sure you choose whichever one is best for you and your lifestyle. But both types of rings contain the same kinds of hormones, estrogen and progestin. I have talked a lot about these in the previous chapters, and how they work, but here's a bit of a refresher. These hormones are synthetic versions of the hormones our bodies produce naturally, and by wearing this ring, you are absorbing the hormones into your body. The hormones work to thicken the cervical mucus and create a barrier to stop the sperm in the vagina. The hormones also bring a halt to ovulation. No sperm movement plus no egg released means no pregnancy.

The NuvaRing

The NuvaRing can last for up to five weeks, but is replaced about once each month. Once you remove the old one, you will replace it with a new one (at the correct time), in order to ensure pregnancy prevention. The NuvaRing and the consistent hormone dosages are also safe and healthy ways to skip your period.

For use of the NuvaRing, there are a few options for you. If you want to get a period, you can either wear the ring for three weeks (21 days), 4 weeks (or 28 days), or five weeks (35 days). Once you choose one of these cycles, when the last day arrives you will take out the NuvaRing and leave it out for seven days. After seven days of being ring-free, it will be time to put in a new one.

For best use, and the easiest tracking, take out your old ring and put in a new one on the same day of the week every time. For example, if you put a new ring in on Monday, then in 3, 4, or 5 weeks you will take it out on a Monday. Then the next Monday you will put in a new one, repeating this cycle. It's alright if you are still spotting or bleeding when your insertion day comes, and you can still use menstrual products like tampons and menstrual cups with the ring in. Just be sure that you don't pull it out with a menstrual cup.

If you want to skip your period while using the NuvaRing, just keep the ring in your vagina the whole time for three to five weeks, swapping it out immediately when it is time. You can do this in one of two ways:

1. Pick a date or day of the month and always remove and replace your ring on that date. So if you choose the third of one month, you'll take it out and replace it right away on the third of every month from then on. Don't worry if some months are longer than others, the ring is effective for up to five weeks.

2. Wear your ring for 21 days (3 weeks), 28 days (4 weeks), or 35 days (5 weeks) then take out your old ring and put in a new one. Change your ring on the same day of the week every time, so if you put your ring in on a Friday, you will switch your ring every 3,4, or 5 weeks on a Friday.

If you are using the ring and choosing to skip your period, you may still experience a bit of spotting during the first few months. This is nothing abnormal or dangerous, it is simply your body getting used to the hormones and not experiencing ovulation.

For the NuvaRing, your likelihood of conceiving increases if you leave the ring out for more than 48 hours (or two days) in a row. So being on top of your tracking methods and keeping it in is highly important.

The Annovera ring

The Annovera ring is a bit different, lasting about a full year (or 13 menstrual cycles). But you don't just leave it in that whole time, there is a little moving around that has to happen to keep it working well. You will put the Annovera ring in your vagina, making sure it is properly placed, and leave it there for 21 days (three weeks),then you will take it out for a full seven days. After that, you put it back in and start the process over again. As I mentioned, keep track of how many times you use it since it is only good for 13 cycles.

You will be much more likely to get pregnant if you don't change your ring or take it out on time, and unfortunately this is a common thing that leads the 99% effectiveness to lower to 91%. As for the Annovera ring, if it is out of your vagina for more than two hours at a time, or even at different times for those 21 days you are supposed to have it in, your risk of getting pregnant is also significantly higher.

Some ways you can keep yourself on top of your birth control ring schedule include: using a period tracking app, setting reminders, marking it on your calendar, or having a partner or friend remind you. It is highly important to use and replace the birth control ring properly and on time, or else the effectiveness drops and increases your chances of getting pregnant.

Proper usage and insertion

Proper use is highly important, so now let's talk about how to properly insert your vaginal birth control ring. It's actually quite easy to insert the ring, but first you need to check the expiration date on the packaging before use. Now wash your hands with soap and water and take the ring out of its packaging.

To insert the birth control ring, wash your ring with unscented soap and water, patting it dry with a clean towel. This will need to be done every time you use the ring. Now squeeze both sides of the ring together and push it deep inside your vagina. You don't need to worry about the exact placement of the ring, just make sure that you can't feel it when you are walking around. If the ring feels uncomfortable, try pushing it deeper into your vagina, and don't worry, it can't get lost or stuck inside you. You can also leave it in for sex and any kind of physical activity. The only differences between the rings are the length of time you can leave them in and when you should replace them.

You can start using the birth control ring, both the NuvaRing and the Annovera ring, at any time of the month and at any stage of your menstrual cycle. But please note that if you put your ring in within the first five days of your cycle (or within the first five days after your period starts) it will be effective right away. Otherwise, it will need to be in your vagina for seven days before it actually starts working to prevent pregnancy. During this time, it is best to use another form of birth control like a condom.

Properly storing your rings is another important way to keep them working well. For NuvaRings you can store them for up to four months, just be sure to keep them at room temperature and away from direct sunlight. After four months, keep your NuvaRing in the refrigerator, you should also always read the directions on the packaging and check the expiration dates.

For the Annovera ring, you can store it in the little case it comes with when it is not in your vagina. Just be sure to keep it at room temperature and away from kids, pets, or anyone who might accidentally know or touch it. Do not keep it in your refrigerator. As long as you use it before the expiration date, your Annovera ring will be active and effective at preventing pregnancy for 13 cycles.

Benefits

The birth control ring is a highly convenient form of birth control that you really don't have to think about once you have it inserted, which is why it appeals to so many people. It is also highly effective and can be left in during sex, without needing another form of contraception. Depending on how you choose to use it and which ring you have, you really only have to think about your contraceptives once or twice a month.

They have also been known to lighten periods and make premenstrual syndrome (PMS) symptoms less intense as well. The hormones in the birth control ring work to make your period easier to predict, and can even stop it all together, which is something some women prefer.

The birth control ring and the hormones it releases actually have other health benefits as well, such as treating and preventing acne, lessening bone thinning, helping cysts in breasts and ovaries, preventing ectopic pregnancies, preventing endometrial and ovarian cancers, and even aiding iron deficiency.

You can also get pregnant right away after stopping the use of the birth control ring, which is something a lot of women look for. This provides you with control over when, how, if, and with whom you get pregnant.

Drawbacks and side effects

Having to stay on schedule and remember to remove and replace the birth control ring is something that some people don't want to deal with, which stops them from getting this contraceptive. It is vitally important to keep it in for a certain amount of time, not take it out for too long, and be sure to put a new one in at the right time, which is more than what some people want to think about.

There can also be some negative side effects that come along with the use of the birth control ring. Most of these go away within two or three months of use after your body gets used to the new hormones. Some side effects include headaches, nausea, changes to your period, sore breasts and breast pain, spotting between periods, and more vaginal wetness.

As I mentioned, these are typically just signs that your body is getting used to the hormones, but if they don't go away within a few months, you should reach out to your health care provider. The birth control ring should also not make you feel sick or uncomfortable, if it does, seek a medical opinion right away.

Key takeaways

- A birth control ring is a hormonal form of contraception that is inserted into your vagina to prevent pregnancy.
- The NuvaRing and the Annovera ring are currently the only two options available, and you can look further into what cycle option works best for your lifestyle.

- Birth control rings are highly effective, and when used properly, they can be up to 99% effective at preventing unwanted pregnancy.
- It is easy to insert and doesn't have too many particularities, just make sure you can't feel it when you move around.
- There are some other health benefits that come along with the birth control rings, including lightening PMS symptoms, helping acne, and preventing endometrial and ovarian cancers.

Chapter 8
Condoms and Dental Dams

Condoms and dental dams are an entirely different form of contraception than the other methods we have discussed in the previous chapters. They are one-time-use barrier methods. This basically just means that you can only use them one time and they work by creating a barrier between you and the person you are engaging in intercourse with. These methods of contraception are not only used to prevent pregnancies but to prevent the spread of sexually transmitted infections (STIs) as well.

External or "male" condoms

Condoms are one of the most widely accessible and used forms of contraception and STI prevention today. Condoms are not only a great option for preventing pregnancies and STIs, but they are also very cost-effective, with the average cost of a single condom being $0.45 in the US and as little as 14p in the UK. Typically, condoms are made of latex, but if you have an allergy to latex, polyurethane condoms are also available. Male condoms are so widely used and available that there are actually *a lot* of different options available to you. They come in a variety of shapes, sizes, colors, and even flavors. The good news here is that you can't really go wrong with your choice, unless you choose the wrong size, of course.

Standard latex condoms are the most common and effective way of preventing pregnancies and sexually transmitted diseases and infections. These are a tried-and-true option because of latex being a nonporous and cheap material. Just be sure to not use an oil-based lubricant like vaseline or lotion, as it will break the condom down and make it less effective. When using a latex condom, it is best to opt for a silicone or water-based lube.

Latex condoms come in an array of different options, in fact there are even glow in the dark condoms available. Along with flavors, ribbed outsides (usually marketed for *her* pleasure), thin options, and even *tingling* options, original condoms can be a great way to spice up your intimate time with your partner.

These options really play off of the fact that condoms don't just need to be used for contraception, they can actually be used as a part of foreplay and can be used for vaginal, oral, and anal sex as well. Conventional condoms can also come with lubrication already applied, making your job of finding the right lube a lot easier. They can come thin or thick, ribbed with texture, or just normal, all of it depending on you and your partner's preferences.

I briefly stated earlier about latex-free condoms being available if you have a latex allergy, and there are a lot of options available to you! There are condoms nowadays that are made from lambskin, nitrile, polyisoprene, and polyurethane, all of which don't contain latex. But don't opt for latex-free options if neither you nor your partner are allergic to latex, as they are more likely to break down or tear. Lambskin condoms, that I just mentioned in passing, are made from the lining of animal intestines. This material often feels more natural for people and can even increase sensitivity, but they are more porous than other options, and they are less effective at preventing sexually transmitted infections.

As great and commonly used as condoms are, there can be some downsides, such as:

- Decreased sensation in the penis
- Can cause a loss of erection
- Could break down, tear, or slip off
- In day-to-day use, they can be used improperly, dropping their success rates to only 87%

Unlike the previously discussed birth control methods, condoms don't require a prescription, making them available to anyone looking to have safe, protected sex. They can be found everywhere, like drugstores, gas stations, public bathrooms, and community centers. They are also one of the few forms of contraception that do not have any side effects, other than the possibility of skin irritation or allergy. Furthermore, since no birth control method is 100% effective, condoms are great for adding another layer of protection.

It has been found that under 50% of high school students were taught how to put on a condom, so this means kids and even adults are simply guessing. This brings the effectiveness down significantly. Here is how you should apply and remove a male, or external, condom:

First thing you should do is check that the condom has not expired and that the packaging and condom itself has no holes or tears in it. If you see it is broken or has been tampered with, just throw it away. If you or your partner have an uncircumcised penis, you can pull back the foreskin prior to placing the condom. To apply the male condom, simply place the condom on the tip of the penis, you can unroll it just a bit to make sure it is going the right way. When you place it on the head of the penis, it should point out, almost like a little hat. From here, hold the tip in place and roll it down the shaft of the penis, all the way to the base, making sure there is a bit of space for air at the end.

When you have finished having sex, the bit of space at the end of the condom should have collected the semen. To remove the condom, simply pull from the base and take it off, it may roll a bit, but should come off easily. Also, be sure to do this away from your partner to avoid spilling semen on them.

Besides latex and non-latex condoms, there are also internal, also known as female, condoms that can be used for both contraception and STI prevention.

Internal or "female" condoms

Female condoms are a newer and less common version of the condom. Unlike conventional condoms, these are internal and are inserted into the vagina. While they look a little different, they are still used as an effective barrier against STIs and sperm entering the uterus. It is a loose, soft pouch that sits loosely inside the vagina. While external condoms need to be tight and fitted, internal condoms do not. It has flexible rings at both ends that hold it in place and line the walls of your vagina, with one being an opening that rests at the entrance of the vagina, this is also used to remove it. They are made from nitrile, a synthetic, non-rubber latex, and are therefore safe for those allergic to traditional latex.

With female condoms, there are a lot fewer options available. They cannot be found at just any drugstore or pharmacy, so you may need to go to a place like Planned Parenthood, a health clinic, or find them online. There are currently only two female condoms that have been approved by the FDA, which are FC1 and FC2. However, the FC1 condom has now been discontinued, and FC2 is currently the only female condom brand with FDA approval in the United States.

These internal condoms come with quite a few advantages and can make sex more enjoyable for both parties while also creating a barrier between the sperm and the uterus. Female condoms can actually be put in up to eight hours before sex and therefore do not interrupt the flow of intercourse. Unlike male condoms, which can fall off if your partner loses their erection, female condoms will still stay in place. They also do not need to be removed immediately after intercourse, meaning you can enjoy the moment together longer.

As with all things, there are a couple of disadvantages, and these are a relatively new form of contraception, so there are still some things you may find yourself not liking. Such as the fact that they make more noise than traditional condoms. They also only come in one size and cost a bit more than conventional external condoms. They also have a possibility of slipping out of place during sex and have a lower success rate of 79%.

During intercourse, it is normal to feel the condom moving around a bit, but just look out for these problems:

- Be sure that your partner's penis goes inside the plastic, not between the plastic piece and your body. It will be useless and ineffective in this case.
- Try not to let the outer ring slip inside your body. If it does and your partner has not ejaculated, you can remove it and reinsert.
- If it slips inside you and your partner has already ejaculated, then you may want to use a form of emergency contraception.

Learning how to insert it is another hurdle some women aren't comfortable with. But I hope these tips help:

- Start by checking the packaging and actual condom for holes and tears. If all is good, feel free to move forward, but if not, throw it away. Remember to not use your nails or teeth to open the package either, as that may break the condom.

- Now you will squeeze the smaller ring (the one that goes inside you) with your thumb and middle finger, inserting the condom into your vagina.
- Use your index finger in the middle of the condom to push it further into the vaginal canal, as far as it will go.
- Check that the larger, open ring is outside of you and open fully, covering the area around the vaginal opening.

To remove it, twist the larger ring that is not inside you before pulling it out to trap the semen inside. When it is closed, you can pull it out and throw it in the trash.

The biggest plus of these condoms is that it gives women greater control of their own sexual health and activity. By not having to depend on the other person to wear a condom, you can have full freedom over contraception and safe sex, which can be liberating!

Please note that you should NOT use both internal and external condoms at the same time, this does not equal double the protection. The friction between the two materials could wear them both down and cause a tear, making them less effective.

What is a dental dam?

A dental dam is a small, thin, and flexible piece of latex or polyurethane that is used during oral sex. This is used to create a barrier between the mouth and the anus or vagina, and just like external and internal condoms, they are built to protect against sexually transmitted infections and to be used just one time. You can purchase dental dams online or in certain pharmacies or drug stores, or they can be made at home with an external or internal condom. Wherever they are purchased ready to use, they are often very affordable, costing $1 to $2.

To make one at home with an external, or male, condom, open the package and check for holes first. Then, take a pair of scissors and trim off the very tip. From here also cut off the rubber base of the condom. Now cut the condom lengthwise, going from the tip to the base, and be very careful to not poke any other holes, otherwise, it will be useless in preventing STIs. You may want to choose an unlubricated condom for this purpose, or you may want to choose a flavored condom as it will be in contact with your mouth.

To use: place the dental dam flat over the vagina or anus. From here, it will need to be held in place by either partner and be thrown away immediately after.

Key takeaways

- External condoms are a tried-and-true form of preventing pregnancy and the spread of sexually transmitted infections, but it is not always effective, especially if you aren't using it right.
- Condoms are cheap and accessible, not requiring a prescription, and can be found at pretty much every store.
- Male condoms come in so many shapes, colors, sizes, flavors, textures, materials, and thicknesses, can come with lube already applied, and can even glow in the dark. There is an option for everyone and their preferences.
- Female condoms are another great option for people who have latex allergies. Though they only come in one size.
- Internal condoms have a lower level of effectiveness but are still a significant barrier between sperm and the uterus.
- Dental dams are not a form of birth control but are a great and cheap way of preventing the spread of STIs in oral sex.

Chapter 9
The Diaphragm and the Cervical Cap

A brief history of the diaphragm

The diaphragm, or at least the idea of them, is actually one of the oldest forms of birth control. The concept of barriers being placed over the cervix as a way of preventing pregnancy has been around since ancient times. Back then, they were pretty creative with the items they used, such as seaweed, partially squeezed lemon halves, oiled paper discs, sponges, and even little balls of opium. But the first *official* cervical cover was created by Friedrich Wilde, a German gynecologist who developed and made customized cervical molds from rubber for women as a form of birth control.

These inventions were brought over to the United States in the 1850s and did extremely well. At least they did until the Comstock laws of the 1870s. This meant that these devices were now labeled as obscene materials and could not be advertised or sent through the mail.

We previously discussed Margaret Sanger and her activism for women's rights to access birth control. She also played a role in bringing diaphragms to the United States. In fact, when she was on a trip to Holland in the 1880s, she heard of these inventions that had been developed in Germany. When she brought them back to the United States and tried educating women about these devices, among others, she was arrested. But that didn't stop her from sharing the information, in fact, she taught the other women in jail how to use them!

Obviously, we know how the rest of the story goes and that they are now available to be freely purchased today, thanks to the work of so many others before us.

How does a diaphragm work?

A diaphragm is a small cup that is inserted into the vagina and fits over the cervix and a bit of the surrounding area inside the vaginal canal. It is to be placed prior to sexual activity and removed soon afterward. These are typically made of silicone and are reusable for several years with proper maintenance. It should always be used with a spermicide (a gel or cream substance that works to kill sperm).

Without the use of spermicide, the diaphragm is around 83% effective, but that percentage goes up if you are using spermicide.

The insertion of the diaphragm might be a little uncomfortable and odd at first, but once you get used to it, putting it in will be easy! Your doctor or nurse can also teach you how to insert it. It may take some practice to get the hang of it, but following these instructions below, those of your health care provider, and reading the instructions on the box can be of great help.

First, start by washing your hands with water and antibacterial soap, you don't want dirt being pushed up your vaginal canal. Next up, take the spermicide and apply it to the cup however, the instructions on the packaging direct. Now you should get into a comfortable position, almost like you are putting in a tampon, menstrual cup, or menstrual disc. You can also squat, lie down, or stand up while placing one foot on the edge of the toilet or bathtub, just do whatever works best for you. Now comes the actual insertion…. Separate the lips of your vulva with your non-dominant hand and squeeze the edges of the disc together, pressing the rims against one another and folding it in half. Push the disc into your vagina, pushing it as far up as it can go, and make sure the edges are completely spread with the dome of the disc facing down. Tuck the edge of the diaphragm behind your pubic bone and now make sure that it has covered your cervix completely. It may seem like a lot, but seriously, practice makes perfect!

You can put your diaphragm with spermicide in up to two hours before you have sex, but any longer than that means the spermicide won't work as well. If intercourse begins more than two hours after you have put it in, just reapply the spermicide before beginning. And if you have sex again before taking it out, apply more spermicide into your vagina before removing it.

Another important direction to note is that you should always leave your diaphragm in for a minimum of six hours after the last time you had sex, just don't forget about it as it shouldn't be left in for over 24 hours. If you do end up having sex again within this timeframe, apply the spermicide again and start the six-hour time window over again.

Taking out your diaphragm is actually far easier than putting it in. Simply reach a finger into your vaginal canal and hook it on the rim of the disc, from here gently pull and remove it from your vagina. When it is removed, there are some things you should do to care for it and ensure that it lasts all those years. Here are some tips on keeping your diaphragm in the best possible condition:

- After removing it, wash it with warm water and unscented soap
- Let it air dry, don't use a towel
- Store your diaphragm in a clean place where it won't be touched or moved. Also, be sure to keep it out of direct sunlight and too much heat.

When purchasing a diaphragm, it is also important to remember that these are not "one size fits all" they come in a plethora of shapes and sizes, just as women do. In order to find the right fit, seek a consultation from a women's healthcare provider.

What is a cervical cap?

At first glance, a diaphragm and a cervical cap look and operate similarly, but the reality is that a diaphragm covers the cervix and the area around it whereas a cervical cap fits snuggly against the cervix. It works quite like a diaphragm and is inserted into the vagina prior to sex as well, covering the cervix so the sperm can't reach the uterus and in order to prevent pregnancy. Currently, the only cervical cap approved for use and sale in the United States is called the FemCap and it needs to be fitted and prescribed by your doctor or other health care provider. The FemCap is also available in the United Kingdom.

Cervical caps resemble what some people call a sailor's hat. They have a wide, circular rim and a dome bowl that dips away from your cervix, rather than toward it, like the diaphragm. There is also a small strap across this dome that is there to help you remove it after you are done using it. While the shape and coverage are a little different from a diaphragm, the other important difference is the length of time for which you can leave it in. The diaphragm should not be left in for over 24 hours, but a cervical cap can actually be left in your vagina for up to two days.

While this professionally fitted cap is quite effective in blocking the sperm from reaching the egg through the cervix, nothing is ever 100%, so many people choose to use spermicide with this product as well. Alone, and used properly, cervical caps are about 86% effective, but that percentage goes up when it is used with spermicide.

Other ways to make your cervical cap effective include:

- Using it every single time you have sex
- Adding more spermicide to your vagina if you have sex again
- Putting your cervical cap in a while before sex, the best-case scenario would be before you even feel aroused
- Using another form of birth control alongside the cervical cap can make both methods more effective. This includes using a condom, practicing the withdrawal method, or even oral birth control pills.

Just as with the diaphragm, using the cervical cap may take some practice and time to get used to using. When you go in to get fitted, your nurse or doctor will show you the basics and give you any extra personalized tips as well. The packaging also comes with instructions on how to insert and remove the cervical cap. Just in case you forget or lose the instructions, here are some directions you may find helpful in learning how to use your cervical cap:

- As always, start by washing your hands thoroughly with soap and water.
- Now, take a quarter teaspoon of spermicide and put it in the domed part of the cup, also spreading some around the rim of the cap.
- With your prepared cervical cap, get into a comfortable position. You can lie down on your bed, sit on a chair, on the toilet, or on the edge of the bathtub. You can also stand with one leg propped up, or squat down, it all depends on what feels best to you.
- Hold the cervical cap in one hand, squeezing the rim of the cap so that it fits into your vaginal canal. Spread the lips of your vulva with your other hand to make the job easier.
- Once it is inside you, the dome facing down, release it, and push it all the way up to your cervix. Now that it is as far as you can push it, use your finger to make sure it has

completely covered your cervix. Without this, it will be useless.

Removing your cervical cap is relatively simple, but can be a little uncomfortable. Caps have a little strap across the dome that covers your cervix. Start by slowly inserting your finger into your vagina and hooking it on the strap (no need to grab onto the rim here). Now pull gently, sliding it down and out of your vaginal canal.

Just as with the diaphragm, make sure to leave your cervical cap in for at least six hours after you have sex to make sure the spermicide works. This will increase your chances of the cap being effective.

Difficulties with diaphragms and cervical caps

As with every form of birth control, there are downsides to using a diaphragm or cervical cap. These methods are most effective when used properly and every single time you have intercourse, which can be hard for some people to do, want to do, or remember. It is a lot more difficult to insert than a condom and may seem a bit more strange in the eyes of others as well.

The first downside that I just mentioned, the best way for these methods to actually be effective in preventing pregnancy is to use them properly every time you have intercourse. If you aren't sure you will be able to, or even want to use your cervical cap or diaphragm every time you have sex, there are plenty of other birth control methods that don't require you to do or insert anything before you have sex such as IUDs, implants, and birth control pills. These forms of birth control also do not protect you against sexually transmitted diseases and infections, so you will probably also have to use a condom alongside this solution. But using a condom on top of another form of birth control means no STIs and even more protection from pregnancy!

As I said, you have to use them every time you have sex, but you also have to use them correctly, which can be difficult for some. Some people have trouble inserting and removing the cap or diaphragm, which can make you even more discouraged in having to use it so often. They also do not work as well if you don't remember the spermicide application, and how often you need to reapply.

Having to use spermicide every time you have sex can be a whole other thing, since there can be side effects that come along with the gel or cream. If you are using this method multiple times each day, it may cause irritation and soreness in your vagina. Talk to your doctor if your cap, diaphragm, or spermicide is causing you discomfort.

Key takeaways

- Diaphragms are one of the oldest and tried-and-true forms of birth control that we still use today.
- Cervical caps and diaphragms are very similar in function, but they are shaped differently and are inserted slightly differently.
- A diaphragm works by covering the cervix and blocking sperm from getting to the uterus. It also covers the surrounding area inside the vagina.
- A cervical cap works in the same way but fits snuggly over the cervix.
- Diaphragms and cervical caps must both be used with spermicide every time they are used in order to successfully prevent unwanted pregnancy.
- Using cervical caps and diaphragms can be complicated, which can discourage some people.
- Cervical caps and diaphragms do not protect against sexually transmitted infections, so if this is a concern for you, please also use a condom.

Chapter 10
The Sponge

The birth control sponge (also known as the sponge, or the contraceptive sponge) is a little, round sponge, just as the name suggests. It is a squishy material, made of soft plastic. To use it, you place it deep inside your vagina, up against your cervix before sex. It covers the opening to the uterus (the cervix) and contains spermicide that also works to kill the sperm before they can reach your womb. Sponges also contain a fabric loop that faces down and makes it easier for you to pull out.

The sponge works to prevent pregnancy in two ways. First, it fits tightly against your cervix, which blocks the entrance to your uterus, so that way sperm won't even make it to the egg. The second way it prevents pregnancy is the fact that it contains spermicide, a gel or cream that kills or slows down sperm before they can keep going to your womb.

It is highly important that you use the sponge correctly and every time you have sex, if this is your chosen method of birth control. Like all forms of birth control, it is most effective when it is used properly and consistently. It is also more effective if you are someone who has not given birth yet.

Women who have never given birth, and who use the sponge every time they have sex, in the correct way, will experience an effectiveness rate of 91%. That means nine out of every 100 women in a year using just the sponge will get pregnant. But the reality is that not everyone will use the sponge properly and every single time they engage in intercourse, as it can be tricky to use at first. That means that realistically the sponge is only 88% effective for these women. Of course, these are the percentages for those who are *just* using the sponge.

But if you are someone who has already given birth, even if you use the sponge properly every time you have intercourse, the effectiveness drops to 80%, though this does not include the use of any other contraceptives. Again, the ideals are not often reality, and the sponge can be hard to figure out or remember to use, so these rates in real life drop to 76%.

The sponge can be used by itself or alongside condoms or another form of birth control in order to make it more effective. Also, since sponges don't protect against sexually transmitted diseases and infections, condoms give that extra bonus of STI protection. You can also use pretty much any other contraceptive method alongside the use of the sponge, such as oral birth control pills, IUDs, and the implant. You could also practice the withdrawal (or pull-out) method, which prevents ejaculation from being inside the vagina. These things will add an extra layer of pregnancy protection.

Some advantages of this method of birth control: First is that there are very few side effects! The spermicide in most of the sponges, if used too often, may cause irritation in the vagina, but that's it for the downsides and side effects. These birth control sponges are also highly cost-effective and cost between $10 and $15 for three sponges (though they are not reusable). They are also very easy to get and you can find them online relatively quickly.

This contraceptive method is not for everyone, here are some things that should suit you and your lifestyle and that you should consider before trying:

- If you would not mind getting pregnant… I know, it sounds crazy. This book is all about pregnancy prevention methods, but the reality is that this isn't the most effective method on its own.
- Be sure that you are comfortable with your body. If you aren't okay with sticking your fingers inside yourself and fidgeting with a sponge deep inside your vaginal canal, this method might not be for you.
- This form of contraception takes discipline to remember, buy more of, and use correctly. If you are not dedicated, it won't be as effective.
- If you are someone who is likely going to have sex more than once, twice, or even three times in 24 hours, one sponge can do the job, it will work however many times you need it to while it's in place. You don't need to remove it and replace it with each round. Just don't take it out right after. You will need to leave it in for a minimum of six hours after the last time you had sex. Also, don't leave it in for longer than 30 hours.
- Allergies are another big thing to mention, if you are allergic to spermicide, sulfa drugs, or polyurethane, then you should not use the birth control sponge.

Now for the big question: *How do I insert the birth control sponge?*

As always, when inserting something into your vagina, wash your hands with soap and water. With clean hands, take the sponge out of its packaging, checking to make sure it hasn't been tampered with. Now, wet the sponge with clean water. While running it under clean water, gently squeeze it until it becomes sudsy. This is imperative, as the spermicide will not activate until it's completely wet. The sponge should be wet and foamy when you go to insert it.

Now get into a comfortable position, like you're going to put in a tampon or menstrual cup. You can stand one foot on a chair or the toilet, squat down, or sit, whatever works best for you. Then you will hold the sponge facing up (the indent at the top and the loop facing down). Now fold the sides upwards, sandwiching the indent and having the fabric loop face out.

When you go to insert the sponge, the folded side needs to face the front of your body, and the fabric loop facing the back of your body. Insert the folded sponge into your body and push it as far as it will go, it will naturally unfold as you push it up. When you let go, it will fully unfold and cover your cervix. Now check that it has been pushed all the way back and remove your fingers.

Long story short: wet the sponge, get in position, fold it, insert it, and make sure it is in the correct position. Insertion will become easier the more you use it.

You can insert the sponge up to 24 hours before you have sex, but remember that it is active as soon as it is inside you. This way, you can have birth control ready before you even have sex, which means no interruptions. You can safely have sex as many times as you want within 24 hours without removing it, just leave it in for at least six hours after the last time before you take it out.

To take the sponge out, just slide a clean finger inside your vagina and hook it onto the fabric loop. You should have no trouble sliding it right out, but if you do, just sit on the toilet and bear down like you are going to the bathroom. From here, throw it right in the trash, don't flush it down the toilet. It is not reusable and is only good for one 24-hour period once it is inside your vagina.

Key takeaways

- The sponge is not for everyone and doesn't have the highest effectiveness rate unless used alongside another form of contraception.
- There are practically no side effects, other than some possible irritation from the spermicide, which is one reason so many people love this method.
- They are not reusable but can be used however many times you want without removing them within a 24-hour period.
- Insertion can feel uncomfortable at first, but with practice, it gets better.
- These sponges are less effective if you are someone who has already given birth, your success rates dropping more than 10%.
- You will need to use a condom in addition to the sponge if you are concerned about sexually transmitted infections, as the sponge does not offer protection from STIs

Chapter 11
Topical Agents

Spermicide

Spermicide is a topical substance that comes in gels, foams, jellies, creams, and sponges that kill sperm on contact and heavily reduce their ability to move. This form of birth control is not typically used on its own and is usually in conjunction with another kind of contraceptive. Though it can reduce the risk of an unwanted pregnancy all by itself.

Just like every form of birth control, it is best used and most effective when used properly and consistently. Read the instructions on the packaging of your specific spermicide to make sure you are doing everything correctly. Otherwise, it may not be as effective. When it comes to the numbers, if used properly, spermicide is 82% effective on its own, but people are not perfect and those numbers drop to 72% effective when in use in the real world. Using spermicide alone isn't the most effective form of preventing pregnancy, but it is definitely better than using nothing at all. If you are serious about not getting pregnant, at least use this alongside the pull-out method.

Spermicide works because it contains an ingredient called Nonoxynol-9. This is what actually kills and slows the sperm down. But it isn't the best form of birth control by a long shot, in fact, it is more of a supplementary form of contraception that is added to sponges, cervical caps, condoms, and diaphragms.

Some benefits of spermicide are that it is easy to use and widely accessible. You also do not need a prescription in order to purchase this form of birth control. Spermicide is highly convenient as well and can actually be used as a part of foreplay if you don't want your contraceptives interfering with the flow of your sex. Additionally, there are no hormonal side effects as spermicides do not contain any hormones.

There are many different forms of spermicide, which means you can choose what is best for you. Here is a list of 5 different types of spermicide and instructions on how to use them:

1. Spermicidal foam

Contraceptive spermicidal foam comes in an aerosol container almost similar to mousse hair styling products. In order to use it, you need to shake it for at least 30 seconds. Then take the tip of the applicator and press the nozzle down. This will then fill the applicator with the contraceptive foam. From here, you can lie down and insert the applicator into your vagina, then push the plunger to release the foam. As soon as the foam is inside you, it is active. Therefore, you should not insert it more than one hour before you have sex. However, best practice would be to insert it no more than thirty minutes prior to intercourse.

After use, wash the applicator with water and unscented, antibacterial soap. Then you can store it in a clean, dry place until you are ready to use it again.

2. Contraceptive film

VCF (vaginal contraceptive film) is a 2-inch by 2-inch sheet of thin film. Actually, it looks and feels similar to wax paper. When it is inside you, it absorbs vaginal secretions and melts away into a thick gel. In this way, it doesn't just kill the sperm upon contact, it also works as a barrier between the sperm and the uterus.

For insertion, make sure your hands are clean and dry. Then fold it in half once, then in half again. Place the folded sheet on the tip of your finger and slowly insert it into your vagina, pushing it deep inside you, preferably on or near the cervix. That is when it will melt away, but you need to wait at least fifteen minutes before having sex so that it can activate and dissolve completely.

You will need to use a new sheet of vaginal contraceptive film each time you have sex and keep in mind that one sheet is only good for up to one hour.

3. Contraceptive inserts, suppositories, or tablets

Contraceptive inserts are a solid version of spermicide that is concentrated on small tablets. These tablets are about a half-inch long and less than a quarter-inch wide. They work by dissolving into a spermicidal foam inside you after insertion.

When you have washed and dried your hands, simply lay down and insert the suppository inside your vagina, as close to your cervix as possible. Wait for 10 to 15 minutes before having sex to allow the tablet to dissolve into a foamy substance and activate. A new tablet should be used every time you have sex and be sure to allow it to fully dissolve before penetration. Each form of these inserts works in about the same way, but you may experience a distinct sensation as they dissolve. Regardless, it is always best to read the instructions before use.

4. Spermicidal jelly

Spermicidal jelly is yet another form of this contraceptive and works in the same ways as the others to prevent pregnancy. This jelly comes in a tube and is typically used by applying it to a cervical cap or diaphragm, but it can still be used on its own.

In order to use it, simply squeeze the tube and push the jelly into the applicator. Then insert it into your vagina. Just be sure to use a second dose if your sexual act lasts longer than one hour or if you have sex more than once, even if it is in less than an hour. But when this is used with a diaphragm or a cervical cap, protection from pregnancy lasts up to six hours.

Another thing that makes spermicidal jelly different from foam, tablets, film, and sponges is that it can also provide a form of lubrication.

5. Spermicidal gels and creams

Spermicidal creams and gels work in the same way as spermicidal jellies and can also provide lubrication as well. But these gels and creams come in different textures and thicknesses. They also are much less likely to drip and make a mess during or after intercourse than other forms of spermicide contraception.

In order to use it, twist the applicator on the end of the tube to fill it with the cream or gel. Now twist off the applicator and insert it into your vagina, close to your cervix. Then press the plunger to release the cream or gel.

This type of spermicide works best when you use it directly before you have sex. Most kinds of gels and creams should not be inserted more than fifteen minutes before you have sex. Though there is one exception called Advantage 24, it is a gel that releases nonoxynol-9 and can provide pregnancy protection for a full 24 hours.

With each one of these forms of spermicide, there will be different options and brands, which means different application types and different instructions. No matter what, you should always read the instructions and follow the direction and recommendations of your healthcare provider.

This over-the-counter form of birth control is a great option for those who aren't completely against getting pregnant or those who want to use it as a supplementary contraceptive. It has nearly no side effects except for the possibility of irritation if used too often or multiple times every day. Speak with your healthcare provider about any concerns or questions you may have and always be sure to let them know if you are experiencing any irritation at all.

It is also important to note that spermicide does not protect against sexually transmitted infections or diseases, therefore, if you don't know the status of your sexual partner, it is best to always use a condom.

Vaginal acidifying gel

Vaginal acidifying gel is another simple and easy-to-use contraceptive option that is quite similar to spermicide, though it works a little differently. It is actually a bit more effective than just spermicide, working at 86% effectiveness. But a prescription is required, and it is not quite as widely available as a typical spermicidal gel, cream, or foam. Another plus for many people, just like with spermicide, there are no hormones and the gel only works by stopping the sperm from moving to the uterus. If you use this, you will still get a period and experience ovulation, and since it is not 100% effective, use of an additional form of contraception is also highly recommended.

So, *what exactly is vaginal acidifying gel?* Vaginal gel is available in the US and the UK under the name Phexxi. It comes in a one-dose only, ready-to-use applicator that has been prefilled with the gel, you can use this up to one hour before you have sex. Vaginal acidifying gel is safe to be used alongside condoms, internal condoms, and diaphragms, and can even be used with spermicide as well, all for extra pregnancy protection.

Vaginal gel works by actually lowering the pH, or increasing the acidity levels, of the vagina. Vaginal acidifying gel contains a mix of lactic acid, citric acid, and potassium bitartrate. This all basically means that the more acidic the environment of the vagina is, the harder it is for the sperm to swim to the egg. This gel works and is active immediately after you insert it into your vagina, and works for up to a full hour, not dripping, leaking, or making a mess and staying inside your vagina throughout sex.

Insertion is quite simple actually, and is used similarly to a tampon. Each applicator comes filled with a full dose, and you need to use the full plunger in order to get the maximum amount of protection from it. As I mentioned, it is active for up to an hour, but if you have sex more than once, you will need to insert more. When you place the tip of the applicator into your vagina, close to your cervix, press the plunger, and release all the gel, easy as that!

Please do note that vaginal acidifying gel does not protect against sexually transmitted diseases and infections. Therefore, you should use a condom every time you engage in intercourse with someone and don't know their testing status.

Key takeaways

- Spermicide works in many forms and you will probably be able to find one that works best for you.
- These are not the most effective forms of birth control and are best used in conjunction with another contraceptive or condom.
- There are no spermicide options that require a prescription, from film to jellies, creams, and tablets, you can get any of these options over the counter, meaning they are some of the most widely available forms of birth control out there.
- Spermicide and vaginal acidifying gel do not protect you against sexually transmitted infections and should only be used for pregnancy prevention.
- Vaginal acidifying gel works by making the vaginal environment more acidic and making it harder for the sperm to swim to the egg. It works even better than most spermicides and can actually be used alongside spermicides to provide extra protection.

Chapter 12
Permanent Contraception and Sterilization

Tubal ligation and female sterilization

Tubal ligation, also known as having your tubes tied or tubal sterilization, is a form of permanent birth control for women. During the procedure for this permanent sterilization, your fallopian tubes are cut, tied, or blocked permanently as a way of preventing pregnancy. Tubal ligation means that the egg can't travel during ovulation from the ovaries to the fallopian tubes. It also blocks the sperm from traveling up to meet the egg, all of which prevents pregnancy very effectively. But it is important to note that just because this blocks the egg doesn't mean it stops your menstrual cycle. You will still get periods. The nice thing is that there are no medications to remember and no extra steps to take prior to sexual activity. Once the procedure is done and healed, you are protected from pregnancy.

Tubal ligation is a procedure that can be done at any time during your menstrual cycle, including directly after childbirth, or paired with another abdominal procedure or surgery, including a C-section. It is also highly important to note that tubal ligation procedures are permanent and generally cannot be reversed. If you want to reverse it, you can try for major surgery, though it really isn't a guarantee that it will be effective.

This is one of the most common forms of long-term or permanent sterilization. It works to permanently prevent pregnancy, meaning that you no longer need to use any other form of contraception. It does not protect against sexually transmitted diseases and infections, though. Tubal ligation is not the right choice for everyone. Just be sure to talk to your doctor in depth about the risks and benefits of the procedure. Your healthcare provider may also recommend and offer other options for long-term and highly effective contraception such as an IUD or the hormonal implant.

Risks of tubal ligation

The procedure for tubal ligation includes an operation that makes two incisions in your abdomen and requires anesthesia. Because it is a surgical procedure, there are some risks involved, which include:

- Potential damage to bowel, bladder, or major blood vessels
- A possible adverse reaction to the anesthesia
- Infection at the sight of the incisions or improper wound healing
- Continued pelvic or abdominal pain after the healing process
- A failed or non-effective procedure, resulting in an unwanted pregnancy
- A rare condition called Post-Tubal Ligation Syndrome that is characterized by hot flashes, irritability, mood swings, menstrual bleeding and cramping

These reactions and risks are not too common, in fact, there are some things you can do that can help lower your chances of experiencing them. Some things that put you at *more* risk include:

- History of failed pelvic or abdominal surgery. Or even history of surgery in that area in general
- Being overweight or obese
- Diabetes

How to prepare and what to expect from the operation

Before you commit to the procedure, your health care provider will talk to you about the different risks and reasons for permanent sterilization. Together, you will talk about potential benefits, risks, and things that might make you regret your decision in the future, this may include young age or a change in marital status. Your healthcare provider will also cover the following details with you beforehand:

- Potential risks and side effects
- The details of the operation
- Causes and the probability of effectiveness of the sterilization
- How you can prevent sexually transmitted diseases and infections
- When it is the best time for your body to receive the procedure

Before the procedure, you may be asked to take a pregnancy test, and are more likely to do so if you have had unprotected sex within the last five days (or 120 hours) just to make sure that you are not pregnant. From here, your doctor will probably brief you one last time on the following details of the operation, that I will go over now.

When you have the procedure, either a needle will be inserted, or a small incision will be made through your belly button so your abdomen can be inflated with a gas, typically carbon dioxide or nitrous oxide. After that, a surgical device called a laparoscope is inserted into your abdomen.

In most cases, your doctor will make a second incision as well and insert special instruments through your abdominal wall. These instruments will then seal your fallopian tubes by destroying parts of the tubes, or clipping them shut with plastic rings or clips.

If you have a tubal ligation surgery directly after childbirth your doctor will make a small incision just below your belly button, which provides easy access to your fallopian tubes, and goes through the same process. If you are going to have a tubal ligation during a C-section, your doctor will just use the incision that was used to deliver your baby.

After the procedure, if gas was used, it will be removed and released. You will be allowed to go home just a few hours after the operation. It is also good to know that having a tubal ligation alongside childbirth doesn't increase the time you need to stay in the hospital after giving birth.

Alongside some discomfort at the site of the incision, you might also experience some abdominal pain or cramping, fatigue, dizziness, bloating, or even shoulder pain. Your healthcare provider will discuss your post-operation plan and how you can care for yourself after the procedure as well.

Vasectomies and male sterilization

A vasectomy is a form of male birth control that works by cutting the supply of sperm to a man's semen and is carried out by sealing the tubes that bring the sperm. This is a very low risk form of contraception and is usually performed under local anesthesia and in an outpatient setting or clinic. It is important to be sure that you don't want to father a child in the future, as this is considered a permanent form of sterilization, even though it can often be surgically reversed.

Male sterilization and vasectomies are a good option for couples and men who are sure that they don't want children in the future. In fact, it is a male birth control method that is practically 100% effective, and is a good option if their partner has had poor reactions to methods of female birth control in the past. It is also a lot more cost effective than female sterilization (tubal ligation) and long-term use of female contraceptives. It also means that there will be no need to interrupt sex to work out a form of contraception or find a condom.

Risks and side effects

As I mentioned, this is a very low risk operation that does not have a lot of potential side effects. A potential risk is that you may change your mind and want to father a child in the future, though if this happens (unlike with tubal ligation) it can usually be reversed if truly needed.

If a man has chronic testicular pain or even testicular disease, he is not a candidate for a vasectomy. But for most men, they experience no noticeable side effects at all.

That being said, potential side effects *directly* after surgery include:

- A blood clot or bleeding inside the scrotum
- A bit of blood in the semen
- Bruising of the scrotum
- Mild pain or discomfort
- Swelling

Misconceptions and unfounded claims surrounding vasectomies

A lot of men have beliefs about vasectomies that are misinformed and have no scientific or evidential backing. Many people unfortunately believe everything they read, see or are told, meaning misinformation gets spread like wildfire. These fears are completely unfounded and should not be a reason for ruling out a vasectomy. Here are a few examples:

- *Will a vasectomy affect sexual performance?*—Getting a vasectomy won't affect your performance, masculinity, or sex drive in any way. It simply works to prevent you from getting someone pregnant. In fact, some men have even reported a higher level of sexual satisfaction after getting a vasectomy. Without the fear of an unwanted pregnancy, this could be a way of loosening up and freeing yourself to be completely present and in the moment with your partner.
- *Will it permanently damage sexual organs?*—There is *very* little risk that the testicles, penis, or reproductive organs will be injured or damaged in the process of receiving a vasectomy. Nothing should go wrong or be damaged if the surgeon is skilled and experienced. Even further, next to no reports have been filed regarding the damage of these sexual organs if you are in good health, a suitable candidate for a vasectomy, and your doctor knows exactly what they are doing.
- *Will it increase the risk for certain cancers?*—Some people are concerned about a potential link between a vasectomy and testicular cancer, though there is no evidence for this and no link has been proven.
- *Will it cause severe pain?*—You may feel a very slight or minor pain, or maybe some tugging or pulling during the surgery, but no severe pain whatsoever. Similarly, after the procedure, there may be some slight pain and aching, but it is nothing to be worried about and should go away within a few days. As always, consult your healthcare provider if you are concerned.

Key takeaways

- Permanent sterilization for women is pretty much nonreversible, and if a reversal is tried it rarely works, meaning it is truly permanent. But it is a highly effective way of preventing unwanted pregnancies.
- A doctor will give you other options for long-term birth control and discuss the risks and drawbacks before you commit.
- You need to be sure that you don't want to birth or father a child in the future when considering these options as they should be permanent.
- A tubal ligation can be performed at any point in your menstrual cycle or even directly after childbirth or during a C-section.
- With female sterilization, you may even opt to get it at the same time as a C-section or after an abdominal operation, making the recovery process easier and the medical process smoother.
- A male sterilization is called a vasectomy and is another form of permanent sterilization. Though there are relatively simple ways of reversing it.
- There are very few risks for vasectomies and most fears surrounding the procedure are not based on evidence.
- Neither of these forms of contraception work to prevent sexually transmitted diseases or infections. This means that you should make sure that both you and your partner have been tested and know your status, or are using a condom each time you have intercourse. Just because condoms can be used primarily for pregnancy prevention does not mean that is their sole purpose.

Chapter 13
Emergency Contraception

What is emergency contraception?

Emergency contraception is a method of birth control that prevents fertilization from occurring AFTER intercourse has already happened. It is typically employed when no birth control has been used or when there is reason to believe that the method of birth control used has failed. Contrary to common belief, none of these emergency contraceptive options will terminate an existing pregnancy, meaning that if the egg has already been fertilized, it will not work to keep the embryo from implanting.

There are plenty of options to suit your situation, and I will go over each of them later in this chapter. But some reasons you may get emergency contraception include:

- You didn't use a condom or any other form of birth control when engaging in sexual intercourse.
- You made a mistake with the birth control that you normally take, such as forgetting to take a pill, change your vaginal ring or birth control patch, or get the shot on time and had vaginal sex.

- The external condom you were using broke or slipped inside you after ejaculation.
- Your partner's penis slipped between the plastic and your vaginal walls.
- Your partner finished and mentioned they could feel your IUD now (meaning it moved).

Emergency contraception typically works by delaying or inhibiting your ovulation and the release of the egg. Again, it will not keep an already fertilized egg from implanting into your uterine lining.

There can be a few side effects, though most of them are specific to the type of emergency contraception you use. They include nausea, headaches, vaginal spotting or bleeding, breast soreness, dizziness, fatigue, and abdominal pain.

Plan B and the morning-after pill

A levonorgestrel pill, morning-after pill, can actually lower your chances of getting pregnant by about 75-90% if you take it within three days of having unprotected sex. These levonorgestrel pills come in a lot of different options, such as Plan B One Step (sold as Levonelle in the United Kingdom), My Way, Take Action, Option 2, AfterPill, Preventeza, Aftera, My Choice, and EContra. You can actually take Plan B and a few other types of these pills up to five days after unprotected sex, but the sooner you take it, the better it will work. The longer you wait, the less effective it will be.

Though there are a lot of different options and brands for morning-after pills, these medicines might not work best for you if you weigh over 165 pounds (or have a body mass index over 30), and in that case, a copper IUD or the Ella pill may be a better choice for you. Also, note that you should not take Plan B or any other type of morning-after pill if you have taken Ella within the last 3 days.

Plan B and morning-after pills are quite safe and there are very few reports of serious problems or side effects from the millions of people who have taken them. Your next period after taking a morning-after pill may be a bit different from what you are used to, but that is totally normal. It may be a little later or earlier, or even be a little heavier, lighter, or more spotty. But it will probably be the same as it always is.

You could end up getting an upset stomach, feel a bit dizzy or lightheaded, or even have sore breasts for a bit after taking the pill. If you vomit within the first two hours of taking the morning-after pill, it will not have been effective and you should take another one.

Getting a Plan B or morning-after pill is very simple and easy. They are found in most drugstores and pharmacies and can typically be purchased by adults over the counter without a prescription. However, sometimes the medicine may be in a case behind the counter at the pharmacy, so in that case, you will have to ask for it from the pharmacist. Regardless, you don't need to show a prescription or in most cases, even an identification card. You can also find morning-after pills in family planning centers, health department clinics, or a local Planned Parenthood clinic (in the United States).

Ella

Ella is another form of emergency contraception that can be taken up to five days after having unprotected sex, though it is always better to take it sooner rather than later. It is actually more effective than Plan B, being the most effective kind of morning-after pill available and working consistently at an effectiveness rate of 85%. But you need a prescription to get it. You should also follow up with a health care provider three weeks after use in order to confirm that it was effective.

Additionally, you should not use more than a single dose of Ella at a time, more pills does not mean more protection, it may just make you feel sick instead. If you need to take another morning-after pill within five days of taking Ella, do not take Plan B or another levonorgestrel morning-after pill, be sure to take Ella.

If you want to use a form of hormonal birth control after the use of Ella as emergency contraception, be sure to wait six days after you last had unprotected sex before starting the new method. If you are breastfeeding and need to use the Ella pill, pump and be sure to throw out the milk for a minimum of 36 hours after taking Ella. Also note that you don't have to pump and throw away your milk with the use of any of the other forms of emergency contraception.

Ella is a simple and safe method of emergency contraception, with no serious problems or side effects reported. As with the other morning-after pills, it is completely normal for your next period to be a little different from the usual, with a different flow or coming a bit earlier or later, don't panic. It isn't very common, but you could end up with an upset stomach after taking Ella, and just like with the others, if you throw up within two hours of taking it you should take another one.

IUDs as emergency contraception

Copper and Hormonal IUDs are actually the most effective form of emergency contraception, just like they are one of the most effective forms of birth control in general. They can work as emergency contraception if you get them inserted within the first five days after having unprotected sex and are great because they will keep you protected from getting pregnant in the future as well, so you won't need to purchase any other types of contraception (normal or emergency).

Getting an IUD lowers your chances of getting pregnant from unprotected sex by up to 99.9%, as long as it is put in within that five-day window. Additionally, unlike most morning-after pills, there is no weight limit, and it won't affect your menstrual cycle as much.

These need to be inserted and administered by a registered doctor or health care provider, making it a bit harder to get than a Plan B pill. But just like the Ella and Plan B pills, you should try to get it as soon as possible after having unprotected sex, meaning it will be even more effective.

Serious issues, side effects, and problems are rare with IUDs, and millions of women have used them as emergency and general contraceptive options. Some have annoying, yet harmless side effects (like a heavier or more irregular period) but that is completely normal and common. As always, if you have any concerns, be sure to mention these to your health care provider.

Key takeaways

- Emergency contraception is to be used when you have unprotected sex or have reason to believe that your form of birth control has failed you.
- There are a lot of different forms of emergency contraception, from Plan B and Ella to hormonal and copper IUDs. Each one works a little differently, so it is always best to consult a health care provider before choosing to use any of them. Not all options are created equal, but there is bound to be one that is right for you.
- Plan B and levonorgestrel morning-after pills are the most common form and can usually be bought without a prescription. These are highly safe, with very few serious problems or side effects having been reported. But the issue is that they are actually the least effective, particularly if you have a higher body weight.

- The Ella pill is quite safe as well, but is even more effective than Plan B and levonorgestrel pills. Though these need a prescription in order to purchase them.
- Intrauterine devices (IUDs) are the most effective form of emergency contraception and can be used for years after. This makes them both greatly effective emergency contraceptives and excellent options for continual use.
- Every option works best within the first five days after having unprotected sex, but it is always best to get them sooner rather than later.

Chapter 14
A Brief Summary of Natural Contraception

Pregnancy has been prevented for thousands of years using a variety of methods, including cycle tracking, the withdrawal method, extended breastfeeding, and herbs. While these methods have been around for millennia, they are not as commonly used in the US and UK as the options we have discussed in previous chapters. In countries where access to medical care is limited, these methods are more common. Effectiveness cannot be guaranteed with any birth control method, and there is limited scientific research about these natural birth control methods. Please discuss with your healthcare provider before attempting any of the following methods.

Natural family planning and fertility awareness

The natural family planning and fertility awareness birth control method is one of the most well-known methods of natural birth control. It doesn't require any hormonal supplements, devices, or pills. With the methods I will mention below, you can easily track your fertility and when in your cycle you are most likely to get pregnant. While this can be used as a form of birth control, it can also be used as a way of trying to get pregnant, so if you are looking for a method that will allow you to plan when, how, or if you get pregnant, this might be a good option for you.

Typically, the ovaries release an egg around the same time every month. As we learned earlier, this is called ovulation. This is when the egg moves through the fallopian tubes and toward the uterus, if it is not fertilized, you will get your monthly menstrual period. This highly fertile period lasts for about six days each month, five days before ovulation and the day of ovulation. The natural family planning techniques here will help you pinpoint that fertile window and let you know when you should not be having sex or be taking extra precautions throughout your menstrual cycle.

You can practice this natural family planning and fertility awareness in a few ways:

- **Rhythm or calendar-based method**—This is one of the oldest and most common ways to utilize natural family planning and fertility awareness as a form of birth control. It is simple and easy and is just based on the calendar. A normal menstrual cycle lasts between 28 and 32 days, and ovulation typically happens on day 14. So this means that you should avoid unprotected sex between days 8 and 19, since that is the time when you are most fertile. Just be sure to ask your doctor how to best use the calendar-based method for your specific cycle. It typically works very well for couples, though it is not for everyone. If your cycle is not predictable or regular, this may not be the best option for you.
- **Basal body temperature (BBT) method**—Our bodies are so amazing at letting us know where we are in our cycles, in fact, your body temperature can rise 0.5 to 1 degree Fahrenheit (or 0.2 to 0.6 degrees Celsius) when you ovulate and stay there until your next menstrual period. If you are going to use this method, you take your temperature before you get out of bed each morning and

before you have anything to eat or drink. Basal body temperature method isn't the best way of preventing pregnancy since it tells you when you have already ovulated, so this is more supplemental for the other natural family planning methods.

- **Cervical mucus or ovulation method**—With this method, you use the consistency of your cervical mucus to track where you are in your menstrual cycle. When you are ovulating, the mucus your cervix produces will be clear, wet, and stretchy, almost like raw egg whites. Just be sure to write down what your mucus looks and feels like each day to track where you are in your cycle and whether you are highly fertile. Talk to your doctor about what each phase of your menstrual cycle looks like in your cervical mucus and how you can pinpoint each of them. Also, do note that this method requires some tracking and a fairly regular cycle to be the most effective.
- **Symptothermal method**—This is basically a method where you combine two natural family planning and fertility awareness methods in order to have an even more effective tracking and birth control method. This is typically done with the cervical mucus and basal body temperature methods or calendar and BBT methods. Any of the above methods can be used together, and simultaneously, and the best part is that overlapping them will not cause any side effects or faults in the contraceptive methods.

Natural family planning isn't for everyone and it is definitely a bit more work than other forms of birth control, but there are a lot of benefits including: no hormones, no devices, that you can stop anytime and that it is completely free. It also follows most religious guidelines and can be used in the opposite manner to help you conceive more easily as well.

Lactational Amenorrhea

The lactational amenorrhea method (LAM) is yet another form of natural birth control and family planning. Producing breast milk is called lactation and not having a period is called amenorrhea, therefore this form of natural contraception gets the name *lactational amenorrhea.* It is a temporary form of contraception that relies on you producing breast milk, or breastfeeding, after giving birth. It is possible to use this form of birth control for up to six months after you give birth if the details and conditions that I list below are followed and met.

This method works exclusively by breastfeeding through the six months after giving birth. This is because the hormones that produce your breastmilk are the same hormones that will stop your ovaries from releasing an egg to be fertilized. For this method to be effective, the following conditions need to be met:

- Your baby must be under 6 months old
- AND you must have not have had a menstrual period since giving birth
- AND the baby needs to be exclusively breastfed. Meaning that breast feeds happen at least every three to four hours throughout the day and every six hours through the night. This means no pumping and no formula, your baby getting nothing but breast milk straight from your chest.

If any of the above conditions are not met or stop being met (such as you getting a period or your baby being over 6 months old or you start feeding them formula) you will need to assume that lactational amenorrhea no longer works for you anymore and you need to start another form of birth control. It is important to remember that pregnancy can occur even before you get your first period after giving birth, since ovulation occurs before a menstrual period.

Besides those risks, this is a very safe and effective method of temporary birth control, being up to 98% effective if all the above conditions are met. Just be sure to talk to your doctor before officially starting this method of family planning.

The pull-out method

The withdrawal, or pull-out, method is a way of naturally preventing pregnancy by keeping the semen away from the vagina. It is highly common and has been used for centuries throughout many cultures and countries. It is exactly what it sounds like: pulling the penis out of the vagina just before ejaculation. If the semen gets into your vagina, there is every chance of getting pregnant, but if not, then you should have a reduced chance of pregnancy. You just need to be sure to be practicing this method before *any* semen comes out in order to best prevent conception and be using this every single time you have vaginal sex.

In order for this method to work best, you need to be sure that your partner is pulling out BEFORE they finish and are ejaculating away from your genitals. If any semen gets on or in your vagina, you have a chance of getting pregnant, even if it is low.

This is actually a *super* effective form of natural contraception when used *perfectly*, but the reality is that slip-ups happen. This means it is best to use this method alongside another (such as family planning, a vaginal ring, condom, spermicide, or a diaphragm). Or even keeping emergency contraception on hand could be useful just in case something happens. But even if this is used perfectly, the self-lubrication that occurs when the penis is aroused produces a bit of sperm, though the risk of pregnancy is still considerably lower.

This could be a good option for you if you are dedicated to using it. Pulling out is a free, reasonably effective, and easily available form of contraception that has no side effects. Just remember that this doesn't protect against all sexually transmitted diseases and infections, so wearing a condom if you aren't sure of the status of your partner is a good idea.

You also need to be sure that you have set the expectation with your partner and that they know their body well enough to pull out in time. Trusting your partner to follow through with this form of contraception is highly important, so if you do not know your sexual partner too well or don't know if they will follow through it is best to use a condom or other form of birth control as well.

Herbs

Herbs and plants as a natural form of birth control are a whole topic worth an entire book, so this section will be minimized to the very basic information. Please be sure to consult a health care professional before using any of these herbs just to be sure they are safe for you and your body because everyone is different. I will go over the herbs that have been used and are tried and true throughout history, just know that there are even more options available to you. This is just to let you know they are out there for you to find.

Some herbs and their uses throughout the centuries include:

Neem—Neem is an herb also known as Indian lilac, nim, white cedar, and a few other names. It works to slow the mobility of the sperm once it is inside the vagina, preventing it from reaching the egg and creating pregnancy. It can be used as a highly effective form of male birth control for up to eight months when Neem oil is injected into the vas deferens (or sperm ducts). It is also nearly 100% effective as a form of female contraception when put inside the vagina. When used inter-vaginally, it is effective for up to a full five hours, no matter how many times you have sex. This makes it the most natural and effective form of spermicide available. There are also preparations of Neem that can be taken orally for the same purpose.

There are many ways to use neem as birth control, be sure to discuss your options and potential side effects with your healthcare provider in order to find the best possible use for you, your situation, and your partner.

Queen Anne's Lace—Queen Anne's Lace is not technically a contraceptive, it does not stop the sperm from moving to the egg and does not stop ovulation. It actually works by preventing the implantation of an already fertilized egg, so is essentially a type of natural emergency contraception. It does not disrupt an already healthy early pregnancy; it works by making the uterus a dangerous environment for the fertilized egg. It isn't exactly a form of abortion, it just shifts the hormones in your own body so the egg can't implant and grow to become a baby. Therefore, it typically aligns with most religious beliefs and instruction. It is taken in three doses, just be sure to talk to your doctor or licensed herbalist before officially choosing this as a form of preventing pregnancy.

Pennyroyal—This is yet another unconventional form of contraception and works as an abortive herb. It has been used for centuries as a way for women to end early pregnancies. While this is found naturally and has been used for so long, it is always best to consult a healthcare professional before use to discuss risks (both physically and emotionally).

Buckwheat—Buckwheat has been used throughout the years as a way of disrupting early pregnancy and as a form of emergency contraception. It too works to prevent implantation and makes the uterus inhospitable if an egg is already fertilized. You can take it as a cup of tea and the only warning here is that some people are allergic to it. Before trying any at home remedies, as always, please talk to your doctor first.

Angelica—Also known as Dong quai, Angelica works by promoting menstruation and thus terminating pregnancy. But it can also be used as a way of postponing your menstrual period, either way it makes your uterus an unsuitable environment for implantation. Use all depends on how and when you want to use it, consult your doctor or licensed herbalist about possible side effects and allergies.

Key takeaways

- There are so many options for natural birth control, though they do require a bit more attention and practice to master.
- Natural family planning and fertility awareness can be done in quite a few ways, and is best used in conjunction with another method. There are no side effects and the same methods can be used to plan a pregnancy in the future.
- Breastfeeding a baby is another way of stopping ovulation and your period for up to six months after giving birth. Meaning that you don't have to go on a hormonal form of contraception soon after giving birth.
- There are also lots of herbs that have been used for centuries to prevent fertilization or implantation of a fertilized egg. These have minimal side effects. Just be sure to discuss your ideas with a health care provider before beginning anything on your own.
- Neem can be used as both a male contraceptive and a female one, meaning that if your male partner is looking for a natural way to prevent pregnancy on their end, it could be a good option. There are also different ways you and your partner can use this contraceptive, from injections and pills to being able to apply the oil vaginally.

- A reminder, however, that none of these methods offer any protection against sexually transmitted infections, so please consider using a condom if you are uncertain of your partner's STI status.

Chapter 15
Outercourse

What is outercourse?

Outercourse is basically sexual activities and pleasure that simply do not include penetrative sex. However, the word *outercourse* often means different things to different people. Some couples might define this as any sexual activity at all that just doesn't involve penis in vagina penetration, some might consider it oral or anal sex. Others may consider oral and anal sex as penetration and not include it in the outercourse category. Regardless, this is up to you and your partner to decide what it means to you, and it really only works as long as there is no vaginal penetration.

Some couples view outercourse as a form of abstinence (or purposefully choosing to not have sex for personal or religious reasons). Others consider it just another form of sex, even though there is no penis in vagina penetration. Although people may disagree with each other's definitions, it doesn't matter, because it is completely up to you for how you want to practice it.

During outercourse, you and your partner may kiss, rub one another, caress, masturbate, use sex toys, or practice oral sex. People also choose to practice outercourse for a variety of different reasons as well, including: not being ready for penetrative sex, penetration not being comfortable or possible, wanting to prevent pregnancy, or to learn more about their partner and their body.

There is no right or wrong way to practice outercourse, but if you are using it as a way to prevent an unwanted pregnancy, it could be a good option for you.

Benefits of outercourse

- It takes the pressure off of penetrative performance— With penetrative sex completely off the table, you and your partner can explore a multitude of other ways to please each other.
- Lowers the risk of conceiving—Because there is no vaginal penetration in outercourse, if done correctly, it means there is no chance for sperm to reach and fertilize your egg. Just be sure that no semen or pre-cum comes in contact with the vulva or vagina, as that means there is a risk of pregnancy.
- It gives you and your partner space to discover what you like—when the assumption that sex automatically equals vaginal penetrative sex is pushed aside; it creates a space for discovery. You and your partner can touch each other more and communicate what you like without vaginal penetration. Discover where you like to be kissed, held, and touched, and figure out where your partner likes those things as well.
- It can soothe stressors—The fact is that there are fewer risks with outercourse than with penis in vagina sex. Being able to enjoy sex without, or with less fear of pregnancy, you can open yourself and your partner up to being mindful and present with the pleasure you are experiencing.

Associated risks of outercourse

- It can be misunderstood—Some people will understand outercourse to be something different from what their partner believes. Communication and understanding are key in navigating the moments where you disagree over what is included in the category of outercourse.
- It doesn't protect against sexually transmitted diseases and infections—Just because ejaculation is not happening inside the vagina or there is no genital touching, hands and mouths can spread STIs as well. Be sure to know the status of your sexual partner and take the proper precautions even if you are just taking part in outercourse.
- It can lead to intercourse—There can be an "accidental" path to intercourse through outercourse, or maybe one partner naturally thinks that it will lead to vaginal penetration. With the heightened emotions that come along with sexual pleasure come risky decisions, so it is best to set boundaries and expectations of what you will participate in with your partner prior to the start of outercourse.
- Risks can be misunderstood—A lot of the time abstinence and outercourse is taught and considered a risk-free option to intercourse, the reality is that it can still spread contact based STIs and STDs, and there can still be a risk of an unwanted pregnancy. It can be less risky than vaginal penetrative sex, but that doesn't mean it is completely risk free.

Key takeaways

- Outercourse means different things to different people, and it is really up to you and your partner to decide what you want to do and take part in.

- When practiced perfectly (meaning no semen touching the vulva or vagina), it means that there is no risk of pregnancy. But people are not perfect, so another form of birth control is also recommended.
- There are so many other benefits to outercourse than just preventing pregnancy. It can be a chance for you and your partner to discover what you both like sexually outside of vaginal penetration.
- But no version of sex can ever be deemed completely "safe" so it is best to set boundaries and expectations beforehand.
- Always be honest and clear with what you do and don't want when taking part in sex, whether it is intercourse or outercourse.
- This is not a completely perfect way of preventing the transmission of sexually transmitted infections because certain STIs are spread through touch.

Chapter 16
Things that DON'T Work

People who are having intercourse naturally know that there is a chance and a risk of an unwanted pregnancy. This is why there are so many different forms of contraception and ways to prevent the sperm from fertilizing your egg or that stop the implantation of an already fertilized egg. But the reality here is that not all forms of birth control are created equal.

We have talked about a lot of options in this book, and a lot of really effective ones. But now it is time to debunk some popular beliefs and ideas of completely ineffective birth control. Many people believe that these work because a friend or family member told them, and they have done no research. The best thing for you and preventing an unwanted pregnancy is to do your research and to talk to a health care professional before trying any method of birth control, regardless of whether or not you need a prescription.

Here are a few highly ineffective "methods" of birth control:

Douching—Vaginal douching in this case refers to washing out the vagina right after sex to remove the sperm and prevent pregnancy. The harsh reality is that this really does not work, since there has already been a chance for the sperm to swim up to your uterus. In fact, it actually increases your chances of getting pregnant, rather than lowering them, by pushing the sperm further up into the vagina and closer to the cervix. Not only does this not prevent pregnancy, it can also irritate your vagina and vulva if used too often. Your vagina is self-cleaning and doesn't need to be douched. Douching unnecessarily can cause rashes, reactions, and discomfort.

Hot baths—It is a myth that heat can lead to sperm not being able to swim up to the uterus and fertilize an egg. Regardless, some men practice taking a hot bath right before sex and soaking their testicles in hot water in order to prevent pregnancy. There is no science or research to prove that this works. Just because someone had sex after a hot bath and didn't get pregnant doesn't mean that it works. Pregnancy doesn't occur every time you have unprotected sex, and that should be kept in mind when trying new methods and swearing by them to others.

Homemade condoms—Some people seem to believe that if they don't have a condom on hand, they can just use a sandwich bag or plastic wrap as a barrier form of contraception. In reality, condoms were specifically created to prevent the transmission of sexually transmitted infections and to prevent pregnancy, and they still aren't 100% effective. Just based on this, it should be obvious that a homemade condom wouldn't work to prevent conception. These DIY "options" won't fit, could easily tear, and may cause a reaction. Just use a real condom.

Having period sex—Though a woman is technically less fertile the first few days of her menstrual period, that doesn't mean you are completely protected from pregnancy. There is always a chance, plus the sperm can live in the vagina for up to five days after having unprotected sex.

The drain out method, or sitting/ standing up—Sitting or standing upright after sex in order to "drain out" the semen and not get pregnant is not a way of preventing pregnancy. Naturally, semen can stay inside you and create a baby, meaning that it is sticky and wants to stay inside your vagina. Even if a little bit drips out when you stand up, there will still be plenty left inside you that can still get you pregnant.

Taking your pill irregularly—If you are taking a birth control pill and miss days but think it's fine to have unprotected sex because you *normally* take them on time, you have a higher chance of conceiving. These pills only work when taken regularly, and even if you miss a few and still don't have a period, you can still get pregnant.

Not updating your IUD, patch, or shot—The suggested timelines for these forms of birth control are there for a reason. You should be sure to keep close track of when your doctor tells you to update and renew your birth control and when to use another method alongside your current one.

Key takeaways

- First off, don't believe everything you hear on the internet or the people around you. You will not get pregnant from every unprotected sexual encounter, but that doesn't mean one of these at home methods is effective.
- Some of these "options" can actually cause irritation, reactions, pain, and discomfort. After all, most of these substances were never meant to be touching your genitals in the first place.
- Douching, hot baths, period sex, homemade condoms, and standing up to drain the semen out are all ineffective. If you are looking to prevent pregnancy, simply reach out to a health care professional for advice.

Final Words

I hope this book has provided you with the knowledge and information about the many forms of birth control methods that have been created and discovered, and *really* work. Not only that, but there are so many options and you get to decide what is right for you and your body. In this modern era, you have more access than ever to planning pregnancy, preventing it, and deciding when or if the time is right for you to have a child.

You are the one in control of your body, pregnancy, and life, and birth control is a way that you can celebrate that!

I do not know your history nor your current situation, but I do know that if more women were aware of the options and resources available, we would feel a whole lot more confident, in control, and powerful. Knowledge is power, it's a fact. But from this moment on, you need to figure out how you are going to use that power. This is your chance to take your contraception into your own hands and now is even more important than ever. I have seen birth control and contraception change lives and bring back hope. Now you have the knowledge to see it firsthand as well.

There are so many methods of birth control now, some of which are proven to be much more effective than others. In fact, there are pregnancy prevention solutions that can be as effective as 99%! These include sterilization, IUDs, implants, and more! If used perfectly, these methods are even more effective.

There are hormonal options, there are pills, there are operations, and there are natural methods. It is now all about figuring out which is best for you and your current situation. Just always be sure to discuss your symptoms and ideas with a licensed healthcare professional.

If you take anything away from this book, I want you to know that you are in charge. I want you to know that you can take the lead in your healthcare and birth control journey and that your body is yours alone.

References

Birth Control - History of Birth Control. (n.d.). Encyclopedia Britannica. Retrieved August 31, 2022, from https://www.britannica.com/science/birth-control/History-of-birth-control

Birth Control Methods & Options | Types of Birth Control. (n.d.). Planned Parenthood. Retrieved August 31, 2022, from https://www.plannedparenthood.org/learn/birth-control

Hatcher, R., Rachel, S., & Zieman, M. *(2022, May). Choices.* Managing Contraception, LLC.

Menstrual Cycle | Office on Women's Health. (n.d.). Retrieved August 31, 2022, from https://www.womenshealth.gov/menstrual-cycle

Menstrual cycle: What's normal, what's not. (2021, April 29). Mayo Clinic. Retrieved August 31, 2022, from https://www.mayoclinic.org/healthy-lifestyle/womens-health/in-depth/menstrual-cycle/art-20047186?reDate=21092022

Raypole, C. (2021, June 28). *From Acacia to IUDs: The History of Birth Control in the United States.* Healthline. Retrieved August 31, 2022, from https://www.healthline.com/health/birth-control/history-of-birth-control